Men'sHealth®

YOUR BODY
IS YOUR
BARBELL

Men'sHealth®

YOUR BODY

IS YOUR

BARBELL

NO GYM. JUST GRAVITY.
BUILD A LEANER, STRONGER,
MORE MUSCULAR YOU IN 28 DAYS!

BJ GADDOUR, cscs
BODYWEIGHT TRAINING EXPERT

RODALE.

Copyright © 2014 by Rodale Inc.

All rights reserved.
Published in the United States by Rodale Books, an imprint of Random House, a division of
Penguin Random House LLC, New York. Simultaneous exclusive direct mail edition published
with the title *Bodyweight Burners* by Rodale Inc.

rodalebooks.com

RODALE and the Plant colophon are registered trademarks of Penguin Random House LLC.

Men's Health is a registered trademark of Rodale Inc.

Library of Congress Cataloging-in-Publication Data is available upon request.

ISBN 978-1-623-36383-3
Ebook ISBN 978-1-623-36384-0

Printed in China

Book design by Laura White
Photographs by Tom MacDonald/Rodale Images

10   9   trade paperback

First Edition

This book is dedicated
to anyone who's ever been underestimated.

Contents

Screw the Gym!

You don't need it.

Bank that membership fee. To shed fat and build a body of rock-solid muscle all you need is, well, you.

I used to own a successful gym in Milwaukee. I helped a lot of people from all walks of life lose weight, get in better shape, and improve their overall health using the exercises, workouts, and nutritional recommendations that you'll find in this book. But one day, I came to the realization that owning a gym was actually doing people more of a disservice over the long haul. You see, my clients' success had one major flaw—it was codependent success. Without my continued support and guidance, most people would not be able to maintain the results they achieved. After all, the business model of a gym is based on retaining members month after month, year after year, not on teaching people how to exercise on their own for the rest of their lives. So I sold my gym in hope of impacting more people and doing a better job of empowering them to take control of their bodies without my being there in person guiding them like a babysitter.

I used to train in gyms myself; that is, until I decided to "screw the gym!" and work out at home using bodyweight exercises. At the gym, I lifted heavy weights. I got big and strong, but I wasn't really fit at all. I wasn't athletic. I did more damage than good: I hurt my knees and had several operations. I'll tell you more about that later, but the point is, I realized that the gym was not doing me any favors. I was tired of people chatting with me while I was working out, even when I had my game face and headphones on, clearly not interested in conversing.

I was so over having to wait for equipment or share space with other people who were slowing me down. I was annoyed by the guys wearing shirts that said PERSONAL TRAINER trying to tell me what to do or asking me to keep the grunting and groaning down because it was distracting the other members. *Screw the gym.* I told myself that from now on, I would only do workouts that I could do anytime, anywhere, whether it be at home or in a hotel room. I decided to drop the weights and start using my body weight.

At first, I had to get over the mental hump that I didn't actually need to be in a gym to get results. I worried that I was going to get weaker, gain body fat, and lose muscle. That never happened. In fact, I got leaner, stronger, and more conditioned. I was also working out more frequently than ever because I could just go downstairs to my little 90-square-foot workout den and start training right away. Screw the gym and the health club. I was way better off without them! I think you'll be, too.

DON'T GO TO THE GYM IF …
you think you need to lift weights to build muscles that show.

DON'T GO TO THE GYM IF …
you think you need to jump on a cardio machine to burn fat and lose weight.

DON'T GO TO THE GYM IF …
you would rather train in the privacy and comfort of your own home.

DON'T GO TO THE GYM IF …
you'd rather save time and money traveling to and from the gym.

DON'T GO TO THE GYM IF …
you have to get less than 8 hours of sleep to make a workout.

DON'T GO TO THE GYM IF …
bad weather gets in the way of your exercising.

DON'T GO TO THE GYM IF …
you can consistently and safely work out on your own without supervision.

DON'T GO TO THE GYM IF …
you don't need the support and accountability of others to get results.

DON'T GO TO THE GYM IF …
you don't have a lot of money to waste.

DON'T GO TO THE GYM IF …
you hate going to the gym.

DO GO TO THE GYM if you want to socialize or get out of the house, require access to a locker room with showers, or need a professional trainer to coach you through every set and rep.

Otherwise, screw the gym. You don't need it, even though it needs you to think that you do. What you now hold in your hands is a blueprint to losing weight without weights and building a better body with nothing but your own body weight. This is a training system you can follow wherever you are so you can break through the shackles of the gym and leave that musky scent behind. Everything you need is here and in you.

All You Need Is You
THE JOURNEY FROM BARBELL TO BODY WEIGHT

"Yo, BJ! You coming to the weight room today?"

Football coach Donald Forti's booming voice bounced off the lockers as I hustled to class during the second semester of eighth grade at University School of Milwaukee in Wisconsin. Everybody called him "Coach." He was a larger-than-life physical education teacher, the high school team's head coach, and he also ran the school's weight room. Coach was a seasoned power lifter and built like a tank. A hot-blooded Italian with dark features and a thick Boston accent, he would have made Sonny Corleone shiver, and he scared the piss out of underclassmen like me.

"Yeah, Coach, I'll be there!"

Coach Forti made it his mission to encourage as many eighth graders as possible to start lifting weights. He was preparing his future teams. And it worked.

Coach had a way about him, a presence that drew you to him. He reminded me of high-energy boxing trainer Mickey Goldmill from the movie *Rocky*. He could be as funny as he was fierce when he was sharing outrageous motivational stories from his younger days. We relished being around him. He brought out the best in us.

That afternoon, I walked up the stairs toward the weight room, hearing the clanking of weights, tasting the sweat and chalk in the air on my tongue. As I stepped through the entrance, I saw big guys who looked like man-beasts to this eighth grader—wearing sweaty yellow-stained shirts and grunting as they hefted heavy barbells.

Coach Forti was there in the middle waiting for me and a few of my buddies for our initial lifting orientation. That day, we learned the big four barbell lifts: the Bench Press, the Hang Clean, the Squat, and the Deadlift. We started with nothing more than the 45-pound bar and some light training plates. But the next morning, I woke up feeling like I had completed 15 rounds with Ivan Drago. I swore I could feel every muscle in my body. I could barely walk to the bathroom. I remember feeling excited to tell Coach how sore I was. And I did when I got to school.

"Ice it!" he said.

"Ice what, Coach?"

"Everything!"

I was hooked. You'll find this hard to believe, but I have never missed a scheduled workout from that day on, not in high school, not in college, not even to this day as a 31-year-old man.

For a pudgy, overweight 14-year-old, that day in the weight room was *the* first time in my life I felt empowered, like I had control over my body. I felt I could build myself into something special. And it all happened because I had a great man willing to mentor me.

What I loved about lifting was that it provided the type of instant gratification I craved as an underestimated kid looking to prove himself. Every time I entered the gym, I could find a way to put a couple extra pounds on the bar or squeeze out a couple more reps. I quickly got stronger, built muscle, became a good football player. I had weight training to thank. I became addicted to that feeling of accomplishment. But it had a downside. I became obsessed with pushing myself to break personal records every time I trained. I was on a mission to become the strongest kid in my school.

Over the years, this took a toll on my body, especially my joints. I routinely sacrificed form (and my joints) to get the results I was looking for. The older kids used to make fun of me for how hard I worked, sometimes imitating me grunting and flailing through certain exercises.

Even Coach Forti noticed. He told me not to push so hard and recommended lowering the weight on the bar. But I kept pushing. At the same time, I was eating fast food and plenty of it. It was a recipe for disaster. I put on a lot of weight. And the combination of my weight and weight lifting hurt my knees like crazy.

By the time I was 17, I had gained more than 100 pounds, ballooning to 275. I wore XXXL shirts and size 44 pants. I had my first knee surgery.

When I saw the picture of me (above), taken

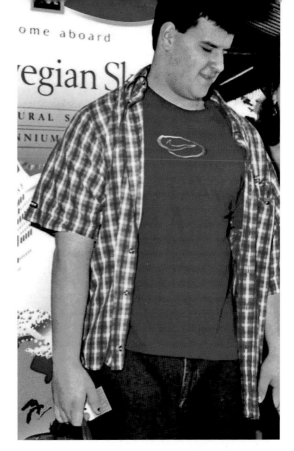

while boarding a cruise ship with my family, I finally realized that I needed to make a change. So I cleaned up my diet, rehabbed my knees, and started running to get in shape. I lost about 50 pounds and played well enough my senior season to be recruited to play football at Amherst College. But just like when I stepped into my high school weight room for the first time, I arrived at Amherst smaller and weaker than the older guys, and it bugged me. I wanted to be the strongest guy again, no matter what. My bad habits returned. I started weight lifting like a maniac and began eating more food than the populations of some developing countries in order to get as big and as strong as I could. I stopped listening to my body and began to push way beyond its limits.

By the time I was a senior in college, I was one of the bigger and stronger kids on my team. I even won our team bench-press contest, lifting 225 pounds for 24 reps (the NFL combine test). I was honored to be selected as a team captain based on my work ethic in the weight room. I truly believed my senior year was going to be the culmination of all of my hard work to date. But it wasn't meant to be.

I tore up my knee in the first week of the preseason. Determined to come back for my final season and be a leader for my team, I got knee surgery and returned to practice after only 12 days and was game ready within just a couple weeks. But my knee wasn't fully healed, and I wasn't the same player. My senior season was a nightmare. I developed an infection in my knee and had to get it drained weekly to get ready to play in each game. I had to be limited in practice, so my conditioning wasn't there. I was a shell of my former self.

In the second-to-last game of the year against Trinity, while jogging off the field during halftime, my knee gave out on me again and I fell face-first on the field. That ended my football career.

At the age of 22, I had had four knee surgeries, and I felt like my body was giving up on me. Where did I go so wrong?

With football done, I started to focus on training to feel better and not worry about how much I weighed or how much I could lift. I also decided to make fitness a career so I could help other people overcome the same issues I had dealt with: excess weight and overuse injuries. I began reading everything health, fitness, and nutrition related that I could get my hands on. I constantly experimented with new training and dietary protocols. I quickly realized that I was strong but not fit. I trained hard, but I didn't train smart. I had muscles, but I was missing mobility. While I could deadlift almost 500 pounds, I couldn't complete one Lunge using a full range of motion without experiencing a sudden stabbing pain in my knees. I could bench almost 400 pounds but couldn't come close to doing a Single-Arm Pushup. I couldn't even lift my own body weight on a pullup bar. How could I have been so stupid as to overlook this?

MY BODY HAS BECOME MY BARBELL—AND AFTER READING THIS, YOU WILL SEE YOUR BODY THIS WAY, TOO.

So, for the first time in my life, I stepped away from the barbell and took a minimalist approach to training. I tried to use as little equipment as possible so I could train at home with no need for a gym membership. I became lean, strong, and nimble. The bodyweight training also helped me program workouts for my boot camps at the gym I used to own in Milwaukee. We promised our clients maximum results with minimum equipment, and that's what they got. I realized how easily I could help other people improve their health and fitness without ever needing to pick up a weight. Most important, I discovered that making progress without pain was actually possible!

Several years later, I sold my gym and launched a start-up called StreamFIT.com that provides streaming fitness videos with a particular emphasis on equipment-free exercises and bodyweight workouts. Now I spend most of my days brainstorming, programming, and testing bodyweight routines that can help our members burn fat, build muscle, and boost metabolism at home or in a hotel room. It's become an obsession.

Fast-forward to today, and I'm now in the best shape of my life. At 31, my knees and other joints feel better than they did before I ever started lifting weights. I can do things now that I could never do when I was lifting weights in a gym. My body has become my barbell—and after reading this book, you will see your body this way, too.

Make no mistake: It is entirely possible to get into peak condition—the best shape of your life—with nothing but your body weight. This book is not an indictment of weight lifting; there's a place for barbells. Rather, it's meant to be a revelation that you don't need to ever pick up a weight again if you don't want to. And if you want to lift weights, that's fine; you can still do so as long as you respect bodyweight training as your foundation.

Open your mind and try these proven methods that have been used for centuries to build the best bodies and create champions of calisthenics. In the end, it is my most sincere hope that you discover that the human body—that *your* body—is the most magnificent machine ever created. You won't need a gym membership, because I'm going to show you everything you'll ever need to know about using your gym within.

But like Coach Forti used to say, "You gotta BELIEVE!"

WHO IS THIS BOOK FOR?

This book is for anyone who wants to get into the best shape of his or her life. You don't have much time on your hands to devote to exercise? This book will show you how to get a total-body workout in 20 minutes or fewer. You're a rank beginner who is intimidated by the idea of trying something new? Don't worry about it. With each of the Bodyweight 8 movements, we start with the most basic move that almost anyone can do; we also show you how to make the exercise easier and harder. The idea is to move forward using baby steps, if you so choose, so that you never get in over your head. You can still achieve an incredible workout using very basic movements and progress when you decide you're ready. Maybe you're barbell phobic. A lot of women feel that they'll turn green and morph into the Incredible Hulk just by picking up a dumbbell. That's not going to happen with bodyweight exercises. These routines will build lean, firm, well-toned muscles, not bulky ones, and target those areas that a lot of women worry about—namely the belly, butt, thighs, and batwings.

Are you the classic weekend warrior who plays Ultimate Frisbee on his days off, takes part in the company softball league, or participates in adventure races or triathlons on weekends? This book will show you how to regain the physical prowess of your youth and allow you to enjoy the activities you love without having to limp around at work popping ibuprofen. You'll improve your game-day performance, too. Maybe you're a full-on competitive athlete. Regardless of your sport, you must first master your body weight to reach your potential on the court, track, road, or field. Bodyweight training represents the foundation of sound human movement. That's why most fitness experts will say you must own your body weight before adding an external load to a given exercise or movement pattern. This book will groove that bodyweight foundation for you. It will show you key bodyweight exercises to add to your weight-lifting routines and sport-specific training along the way. Done correctly, bodyweight movements will bulletproof your body and reduce the risk of injuries from competitive athletics. You say you already feel beat up? When you walk, you generate enough clicking, cracking, and crunching to put on an instrumental performance at a concert hall? Bodyweight training is perfect because it can help rehab you. Not only is it easier on your joints than using weights and machines but it will make your joints stronger, more stable, and a lot more supple. You'll gain mobility in your hips, ankles, and upper back, and you'll dramatically improve your posture. You'll end every workout feeling better than you did before you started, and, gradually, we'll keep trading that pain for pleasure.

Finally, this book is also for the gamer, the athlete who's already in top physical shape but who wants to take his or her physique, strength, or endurance to the next level. Build your own workout from the superhero-level exercises and add a few extreme progressions. I guarantee that you'll be sucking wind and begging your mama for a glass of water and your blankie.

What's Inside

Here's a highlight reel so you know exactly what you're getting into.

BODYWEIGHT 8 EXERCISES

This is the main body of the book. It teaches you how to master the eight key exercises you need to get in great shape with your body weight. Use them to carve a killer core, sculpt striking symmetry, and build a perfectly proportioned physique. Each exercise has five increasingly challenging levels that take you from ground zero to superhero. The main moves are:

1. **Hip Thrust** (page 46)
2. **Pushup** (page 64)
3. **Deep Squat** (page 82)
4. **Row** (page 98)
5. **Hip Hinge** (page 116)
6. **Handstand Pushup** (page 134)
7. **Single-Leg Squat** (page 152)
8. **Pullup** (page 170)

BODYWEIGHT BURNERS TRANSFORMA-TION PROGRAM

This is a comprehensive five-phase fat-loss program using the Bodyweight 8 exercises that's designed to get you into the best shape of your life in 5 months. What? Five months is too long? Don't worry. After 4 weeks, you will have lost enough weight and become much fitter so that the exercises will actually be easier and more enjoyable to do. You're going to love the workouts and the way you look and feel, and that'll motivate you to keep on keeping on. If you want to follow a structured training plan that tells you exactly what to do when, then this is the perfect workout for you.

BODYWEIGHT 8 WORKOUTS

These are the top eight custom bodyweight workout templates for a variety of goals, schedules, and fitness levels. If you already exercise regularly, have a good knowledge of fitness in general, or have completed the Bodyweight Burners program, then these workouts are the perfect fit for you.

1. **Bodyweight Builders** (page 202)
2. **The Minimalist** (page 204)
3. **Pure Power** (page 206)
4. **Super Strength** (page 208)
5. **Extreme Endurance** (page 210)
6. **The 8-Minute Workout** (page 212)
7. **Ultimate Upper and Lower Workouts** (page 214)
8. **The Shredder** (page 216)

THE BURPEES

The one bodyweight move to rule them all is the Burpee because it works every muscle in your body from head to toe and burns more calories per minute than any other exercise. But you must learn how to do it right or else! Learn how to perform the Burpee with perfect form, learn the Backward Burpee, and try the Burpee Workout from Hell!

BODYWEIGHT 8 CARDIO EXERCISES

These are the eight best bodyweight exercises to hike up your heart rate and crush calories so you'll never need to use a cardio machine again (if you don't want to):

1. **Jumping Jack** (page 242)
2. **Skater Jump** (page 244)
3. **Skier Swing** (page 246)
4. **Sprinter** (page 248)
5. **Mountain Climber** (page 250)
6. **Donkey Kick** (page 252)
7. **Break-Dancer** (page 254)
8. **Chop** (page 256)

THE ULTIMATE BODYWEIGHT CARDIO WORKOUT

This 20-minute weight-loss workout combines the Bodyweight 8 Cardio exercises into one delicious calorie-killing concoction you can do at home or in a hotel room. You can also perform this on the days between your Bodyweight Burners workouts for more rapid results. Go to pages 258–259 to get your cardio on.

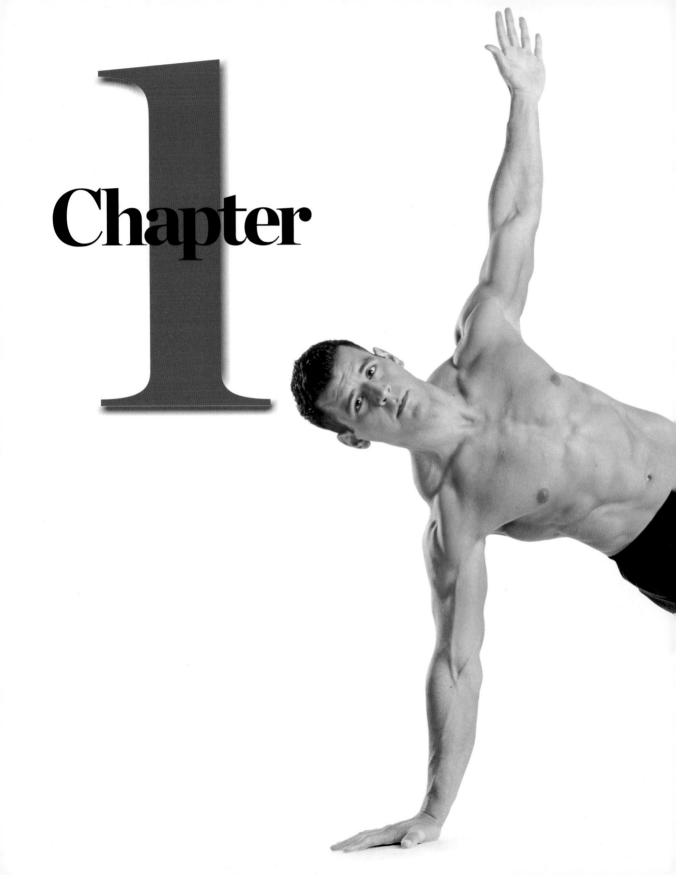

Chapter 1

YOU VERSUS GRAVITY

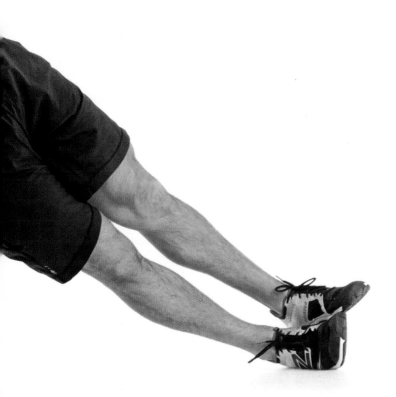

The fitness industry is filled with gimmicks and gadgets, scams and unrealistic promises. Just take a cruise through your neighborhood on a Saturday morning and you'll see the detritus of unrealized weight-loss dreams in yard sales peppered with abs machines and other lonely, little-used fitness equipment at bargain-basement prices.

The stuff doesn't work.

Or the people who bought it didn't know how to use it properly or eat right during training.

Or they simply lost motivation after the first week it was out of the box.

You'll find no such bull between the covers of this book, no wacky claims or suspect fitness gadgets. It's a garbage-free zone. In fact, it's pretty much an equipment-free zone. This book is all about getting back to the basics by using tried and proven bodyweight training tactics to get you moving, feeling, and looking better. It's about taking the time to establish a sound fitness foundation that you can build on for the rest of your life using natural exercises you can do wherever you happen to be. It's about you versus gravity. When you think about it, exercise machines—even old-school bar-bells and dumbbells—are relatively recent inventions. They became mainstream only after the golden age of bodybuilding in the 1960s and '70s. In contrast, human beings have been using their body weight (and formal calisthenics) to be strong and fit for centuries. In society's constant quest to evolve and innovate, we sometimes overlook the brilliance in simplicity.

This book promises results through logic and simplicity. Machines and weights have their place, but just consider all of the incredible benefits to be had by training with nothing more than what God gave you.

THE TOP 10 BENEFITS OF BODYWEIGHT TRAINING

1
Bodyweight Training Can Be Done Anywhere

I like to call bodyweight training "a zero-excuse fitness experience" because it eliminates so many of those common excuses for why you can't exercise today.

Consider this study from Marquette University in Milwaukee, which surveyed 1,044 college students to measure the motives and barriers to exercise. The top excuses students gave for blowing off exercise: lack of time, lack of energy, dislike of exercising in public, facility limitations, and lack of knowledge about how to use fitness equipment.

Bodyweight training vaporizes all of those excuses. A bodyweight workout doesn't cost you a penny. When you use your body for resistance, you don't need to join a gym and feel intimidated about working out in front of angry dudes wearing sweat-stained Megadeth T-shirts. Most bodyweight exercises can be performed in a 6-by-6-square-foot space (basically the length of your body) anywhere, including the privacy of your own home. You don't have to waste time and gasoline driving someplace to work out. Wherever you are—home, work, vacation, business travel—that's your workout facility, and you can keep up with your training without skipping a beat.

All this leads to a related point about anywhere, anytime training. Bodyweight workouts are sustainable. In other words, they are easy to stick with and do for the rest of your life. I believe that if something isn't sustainable, it's questionable, especially when it comes to scheduling workouts or committing to a diet plan. What's the point of doing something for 30 or 90 days if you know that there's no way you're going to keep doing it on day 31 or 91 and beyond? Unfortunately, when most people start a fitness program, they rarely take a look at the big picture. Nor do they consider what's next after completing the program.

Bodyweight training is easy to sustain because it eliminates opportunities to say, "That's a hassle, and I'm done."

In my years of training people, I've discovered three simple truths.

❶ **Most people can commit to high-intensity exercise several times per week.**

❷ **Most people can find at least 10 minutes and up to 30 minutes to squeeze in a challenging workout.**

❸ **Most people can commit to doing some low-intensity activity every day.**

But here's the key: The exercise has to be ultraconvenient, and that's the big plus for bodyweight exercise and what makes it easy to sustain for the long haul.

2
Bodyweight Training Is Efficient

When you train with weights and machines, you often have to adjust the loads during your workout, and that takes time. Whether it's sticking the pin through a different hole in a weight stack, adding weight plates to a barbell, or grabbing a new pair of dumbbells, you lose precious moments while changing weights instead of burning fat, torching calories, and building muscle. Bodyweight exercise significantly reduces transition time, allowing you to seamlessly make an exercise easier or harder or switch between exercises quickly for shorter rest periods between sets, resulting in greater overall training density. The greater your training density—that is, the amount of work you complete in a certain period of time—the leaner and stronger you will be.

Plus, remember that when working out at a gym, you often have to wait for machines to open up or for other lifters to finish with the set of dumbbells you need. There's no waiting game with bodyweight exercises.

3 Bodyweight Training Broils Body Fat

The best exercises for fat loss are resistance-training moves that:

- Work multiple muscle groups at once.
- Allow you to easily alternate between exercises that work different parts of your body.
- Can be made easier midset to allow you to keep working without stopping and resting.
- Can be done anytime, anywhere with minimal space and equipment.

The Bodyweight 8 exercises featured in this book hit these criteria.

The best way to do these exercises for maximum fat loss is to use alternating set formats with minimal to no rest between movements. Short rest periods, typically 30 seconds or fewer, release key fat-burning hormones like growth hormone while allowing you to burn more calories per minute. This approach is known as metabolic resistance training because it provides the maximum body-fat-broiling effect in minimal time, boosts cardiovascular conditioning, and delivers a postworkout afterburn that can elevate your metabolic rate for several days after completing your workout. There are several ways to set up alternating sets.

SUPERSETS
Alternate between two exercises.

TRISETS
Alternate between three exercises.

CIRCUITS
Alternate between four or more exercises.

All these options act like kryptonite to belly fat because they keep your heart rate up the whole time. It's like getting the same aerobic benefits as running but with the added muscle-building benefits of resistance training.

A study reported in April 2010 in the *Journal of Strength and Conditioning Research* showed that alternating between two opposing muscle groups (such as biceps and triceps or chest and back) burned roughly 30 percent more calories per minute than traditional straight sets of the same exercise. There was also a greater increase in postworkout metabolism. Try it yourself: Alternate between Pushups and Pullups without rest instead of just doing consecutive sets of Pushups with rest periods in between. These supersets allow you to do more work in less time. Another way to superset is by alternating between upper- and lower-body exercises or even unilateral exercises of the same movement like Lunges on your left and right leg.

Bodyweight circuit training boosts postworkout fat burn, too. In a study published by the American College of Sports Medicine, researchers constructed a 12-station circuit of alternating upper- and lower-body exercises in which participants performed 30 seconds of work for each move with only 10 seconds of rest between them. The circuit lasted 7 minutes and was completed two or three times for a full workout duration of only 14 to 21 minutes. Results showed that this type of training was ideal for busy people looking to burn fat, build muscle, boost cardio conditioning, and even improve key health markers like insulin sensitivity.

The featured fat-frying workout in this book, the Bodyweight Burners, incorporates this metabolic-resistance-training approach to help you get leaner and fitter faster than you ever thought possible.

4 Bodyweight Training Builds Brawn and Trains Your Brain

Where machines simply train your muscles, bodyweight exercises build brawn and train your brain. Exercise machines were created in an attempt to better target and isolate a given muscle group. They were created to simplify exercises to the point that all you had to do was sit down, select a weight, and perform a set movement on a predetermined, fixed path. Machines were made to be foolproof, so that even a caveman could do it. While this certainly made exercising easier (and sexier), and it certainly helped gyms sell more memberships, ultimately this trend didn't invite your brain to the fitness party.

Consider the Lat-Pulldown machine. When you perform a machine Lat-Pull, because the movement is set by the rigid structure of the machine, all of your body's key joint stabilizers don't need to activate to help you safely execute the movement. The machine compensates for your joints by taking your central nervous system (your brain) out of the equation. You don't really learn the movement but simply go through the motions. So even though you get a big muscle pump and it will burn oh so good, there is virtually no functional carryover to real-world movements. Plus, because you don't train your muscles to stabilize your joints in free space, you increase the risk of injury both during day-to-day activities and in sports. You end up being all show and no go.

Now, let's take a look at the Chinup, the bodyweight alternative to the machine Lat-Pull. With your body as your barbell, your brain needs to communicate with your muscles to execute the movement with perfect form through your natural, pain-free range of motion. Yeah, there's a lot more going on in this bodyweight exercise, and your central nervous system is called into play every step of the way. What's more, because your body is basically flopping around underneath your grip on the bar, the Chinup activates a greater number of muscles.

SECRET WEAPON FOR WEIGHT LOSS
THE PUSHUP

Bodyweight exercises are so effective against body fat that your Pushup skills may predict your success at keeping the weight off. A Canadian study reported in *Medicine & Science in Sports & Exercise* traced the relationship between musculoskeletal fitness and weight gain in a group of individuals for 20 years. Researchers found that the number of Pushups a person could complete (one of the measures of musculoskeletal fitness) was significantly related to how fat they would become over the years. It turned out that individuals who performed poorly in a Pushup test were 78 percent more likely to gain 20 pounds over the next 2 decades. The authors attributed this connection to the fact that those who excel at Pushups are probably more likely to engage in other bodyweight activities that burn fat.

Researchers at James Cook University in Australia compared muscle activation in subjects doing both Chinups and Lat Pulldowns and found that the Chinup required far more work from the biceps and spinal erectors than the lat-machine exercises because of the instability created by the bodyweight exercise.

5 Bodyweight Exercise Prepares You for Life

Bodyweight movements are natural, functional, and athletic. They ready your body for the way it'll be used every day. They teach you how to properly sit down into a chair and build the strength and coordination to help you stand back up. That might not seem like something you need to practice doing now, but how about when you are 87? You'll be glad you did them. Bodyweight exercises prepare your body for going up and down staircases and hills. They'll improve your reaction time to catch yourself when you trip and prevent you from doing a face-plant. They'll make you better at sports while developing all 639 muscles in your body to their fullest potential. Now you've got show *and* go! By focusing on movements instead of specific muscle groups, you develop the entire neuromuscular system, not just your muscles. You develop better overall body awareness and coordination.

Bodyweight exercises are more dynamic than barbell lifts and machine exercises. They warm the muscles and prepare them for action while they strengthen and tone. A study published in the *Journal of Strength and Conditioning Research* found that cadets at the US Military Academy who performed such bodyweight exercises as Squats, Pushups, and Lunges sprinted faster, jumped higher, and threw harder than those who did a static warmup. Why? Study coauthor Danny McMillian says that dynamic moves trigger nervous-system activity, allowing more muscle fibers to be engaged for action. Other studies show that dynamic bodyweight exercises result in more coordinated and forceful muscle contractions.

6 Bodyweight Training Is for Beginners and Experts

One of the biggest myths in fitness is that you can't build serious strength or significant muscle mass with bodyweight exercises. The fact is that all your body knows is time and tension. *Time* describes how long the muscles are placed under a given tension, and *tension* describes the amount of muscular force that is required to execute a given movement or hold a certain position. Though most people think that the only way to get super strong and muscular is to do heavy weight training, all you need to do is select intense-enough movements that require you to create maximal force and activate more muscle fibers. It's the unique combination of high-tension exercises and sufficient training volume (amount of work or sets/reps completed) that is the key to building strength and muscle, regardless of whether the exercise is equipment based or equipment free.

Now, if all you do is the same floor Pushup for as many reps as you can over and over again, like most people do when it comes to bodyweight training, then you will never build serious strength or muscle. That's because you're not increasing the relative intensity of the exercise, you're just adding volume. So, yeah, doing endless reps of Pushups will not help you build as much strength and size as heavy Bench Presses for 5 to 10 reps. But selecting a Pushup variation (like a Feet-Elevated Pushup or a Single-Arm Pushup) that sufficiently challenges you for that same 5 to 10 reps will get you to your strength and size goals. As with any type of training, you must constantly push yourself with more challenging bodyweight exercises in order to progress. Greater intensity produces greater results. (For real-world proof that bodyweight exercise alone can develop strength and amazing physiques, look at gymnasts who perform feats of strength with nothing but their bodies on rings, parallel bars, and pommel horses.)

The beauty of bodyweight training is that it doesn't require any equipment to start, and the basic moves are the perfect place for beginners, women, and endurance athletes who may not have had much strength-training experience. But that's not to say that bodyweight training is only for novices. When you progress like a pro, as I'll show you in Chapter 3, you'll be able to make any exercise harder or easier based on your goals. Whether you're using harder movements for fewer reps to develop strength and boost muscle mass or easier movements for higher reps to accelerate fat loss and improve your conditioning, your body is the only tool you'll need to get the job done.

7 Bodyweight Training Is Fun and Full of Variety

The fun in training comes with consistent progress and always having something special to shoot for. There's no denying the instant gratification that comes with using heavier weights in the gym, but I'd argue that you can use bodyweight training to get the same level of satisfaction and more. That's because the pursuit of overcoming gravity is an endless one.

Lots of people can do a regular Pushup, but how many people do you know who can do a Single-Arm Handstand Pushup? At the time I wrote this book, I knew I couldn't, though it's one of my goals, and I'm working on it. There are literally dozens of small wins and progressions that come in between the basic Pushup and the most advanced Pushup on the planet. These freakish fitness feats will take years of dedicated practice to achieve. But I'm a firm believer that the greater the challenge, the greater the reward. Plus, with bodyweight

training, you're always striving to perform more advanced skills—skills that apply in the real world and that you can show off to your friends and family—where with weight training, you're just trying to keep adding more weight to the bar.

The fun in training also comes with variety. There are hundreds of different ways to perform every key movement in this book using the progression principles that I will teach you: loading, stability, body angle, tempo, range of motion, complexity, and metabolic demand. There are hundreds of ways to construct workouts using these same exercises based on your fitness level, goal, and schedule. Progressive bodyweight training kicks boredom to the curb and will help you bust through any potential fitness plateau. In the end, bodyweight training provides a sound training system that you can use for the rest of your life without ever repeating the same workout (if you don't want to). The options are endless. You'll never get bored.

8 Bodyweight Training Builds Balance and Prevents Injury

Sound bodyweight training builds structural balance—that is, a well-balanced body where the muscles on the front of you are in proportion with those on your back side. You achieve structural balance by paying an equal amount of attention to pushing and pulling movements for the upper body and knee- and hip-dominant movements for the lower body. Unfortunately, our sedentary, seated lifestyles combined with the fact that most people prioritize their mirror muscles (those on the front side of the body) have led to structural imbalances that negatively affect our posture, change our bone and joint positioning, and cause movement that leads to pain.

Too much pushing without enough pulling results in rounded, forward shoulders and hunchback posture, which cause shoulder pain.

A study from Nova Southeastern University found that weight lifters, especially those who did behind-the-neck Presses, were more likely to suffer shoulder injuries due to muscle imbalances. The researchers found that weight lifters were likely to focus on the deltoids, upper trapezius, and internal rotators (i.e., pecs and lats), missing the shoulder external rotator and lower trapezius. This creates an imbalance and decreases mobility, putting weight lifters at a higher risk for injury.

Too much squatting without enough bridging or hip hinging results in quad dominance, weak glutes and hamstrings, tight hips, and ultimately knee pain. Consider the issue of imbalances between your two quad muscles: the vastus medialis and the vastus lateralis. A study from the *British Journal of Sports Medicine* estimates that 25 percent of the general population and 60 percent of the athletic population suffer from knee pain where imbalance between these two muscles is a key contributing factor. And yet there's an easy fix for this: namely, the bodyweight Lunge. A study in the *Journal of Strength and Conditioning Research* suggests that Lunges, which target the inner and outer thigh equally, can correct the imbalance.

It's worth mentioning that you can't just train your upper body and neglect your lower body, and vice versa, as that will also result in structural imbalance. After all, the vast majority of your muscle mass and metabolic potential resides in your lower half, so if you don't pay equal attention to your legs and hips, you'll never get as lean as you can be. In addition, all athletic movements are driven through your hips, and that's why I always stress to clients that it's all about the glutes! Being top heavy will affect your posture and balance and cause pain in your back and lower body. Spend at least an equal amount of time or more on your lower body if you want to be truly fit and injury free.

Bodyweight training also bulletproofs your joints by taking them through full ranges of motion. In particular, it develops strength and stability at extreme joint angles, like full flexion or extension, where most injuries occur. For example, the king of lower-body bodyweight exercises is the Pistol Squat. It requires you to stand on one leg with the other leg extended out in front of your body as you squat down until your hamstring rests on the calf of your supporting leg, and then hold this position with ease before standing all the way back up. To accomplish this feat, you need the perfect combination of strength, mobility, and stability. Once you can do it, you'll have an elite level of athleticism that most professional athletes can't display.

9 Bodyweight Training Strengthens Your Core and Unloads Your Spine

One of the most unique aspects of bodyweight training is that every key exercise is extremely core intensive and targets your abs way more than the machine or barbell alternatives for that same movement.

Pushups beat barbell Bench Presses and machine Chest Presses because your back is unsupported and all of your muscles surrounding your hips and trunk need to kick in to stabilize your spine and prevent your lower back from hyperextending. In fact, a Mayo Clinic study found that Planks, specifically Side Planks, are effective at building abs without stressing your spine. The aligned spine throughout the exercise reduces injuries without sacrificing increasing abs strength. As you progress to more advanced Pushups by narrowing your base of support and reducing points of contact with the ground, all of the muscles between your hips and shoulders need to work together to prevent spinal extension and rotation in multiple planes of motion. Many top fitness experts agree that if you can perform a Single-Arm Pushup, you have all the core strength you'll ever need.

Bodyweight Squats are much easier on your spine than barbell Squats and machine Leg Presses. These heavy external loads put a ton of compressive forces through your spine, and ultimately your lower back is the limiting factor in how much you can lift. A study from the *American Journal of Sports Medicine* found that when performing a weighted Squat with 60 percent of their body weight, lifters hyperextended their lumbar spines, risking serious injury. With a bodyweight Squat, you can progress to staggered and split-stance foot positions to shift the weight more to one leg or the other. This provides the necessary strength and muscle-building stimulus without adding additional stress to your spine. Ultimately, you'll build up to the Pistol Squat, which has you squatting your entire body weight on one leg with no excessive forces on your spine. Plus, single-leg-stance exercises require all of the muscles on the inside and outside of your trunk and hips to activate and stabilize your knees and spine.

Pullups trump barbell Bent-Over Rows and machine Pulldowns for multiple reasons. One, hanging from a bar decompresses your spine and lengthens your body. This is critical, considering that we put compressional forces on our spine all day as we sit, walk, and stand. Two, any time your arms are overhead, your core has to work harder to stabilize your spine. Even if you can't do Pullups right away, the bodyweight Row will still beat the barbell Bent-Over Row because it puts your spine in a safer position while working the entire back side of your body. Though Pulldowns require you to place your arms overhead, they also have you sitting down, often with your knees anchored to the unit, providing you with more stability and leverage to perform the movement, ultimately letting your abs take a break. When you perform Pullups the way I teach them in this book, from a hollow-body position with the legs fully extended, you will be amazed how sore your core will be the next day.

10 Bodyweight Training Sculpts Striking Symmetry and a Perfectly Proportioned Physique

Looking good is one of the most powerful motivators when it comes to working out with consistency. Sure, you want to move better and feel better, be healthy, and have energy to attack life with vigor, but being a lean, mean fitness machine does a hell of a lot for your self-esteem and confidence. Though any integrated exercise and nutrition program can improve your looks, there is no better solution than bodyweight training to maximize your genetic potential—to develop the most natural, aesthetically pleasing physique possible.

You won't look supernatural, you'll look super *and* natural. Rather than resembling a hulking beast that takes up too much space or some weirdly proportioned Picasso painting, you'll appear as a ripped warrior who can move with grace. Bodyweight training has been used to build some of the most attractive physiques the world has ever seen in gymnasts, boxers, mixed martial artists, soldiers, and the great warriors of centuries past. You'll sculpt the shoulders of a superhero, making your waist look smaller from every angle. You'll develop legs of steel, making you as athletic as you appear. You'll forge a firm and fierce midsection, making you a target for endless questions like:

> *"How many hours do you work out per day to look like that?"*
> *"I take it you haven't eaten a carb in the last decade, right?"*
> *"Are you Photoshopped?"*

Bodyweight training will turn you into a Greco-Roman statue. Men, you'll sculpt striking symmetry and a perfectly proportioned physique. Ladies, you'll carve a classically beautiful physique and a flawless figure. You will look the best you possibly can. You will look timeless.

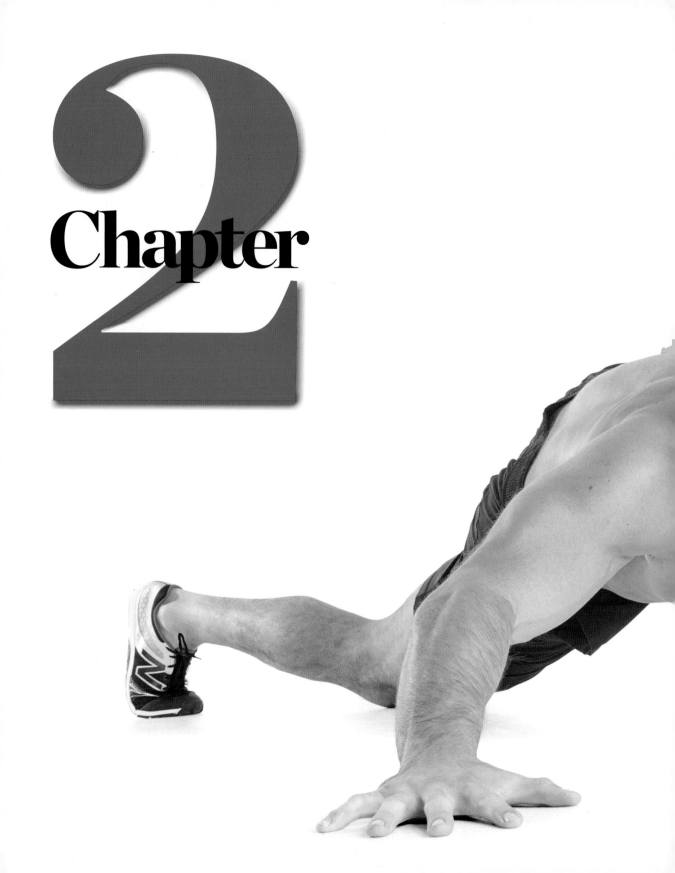

Chapter 2

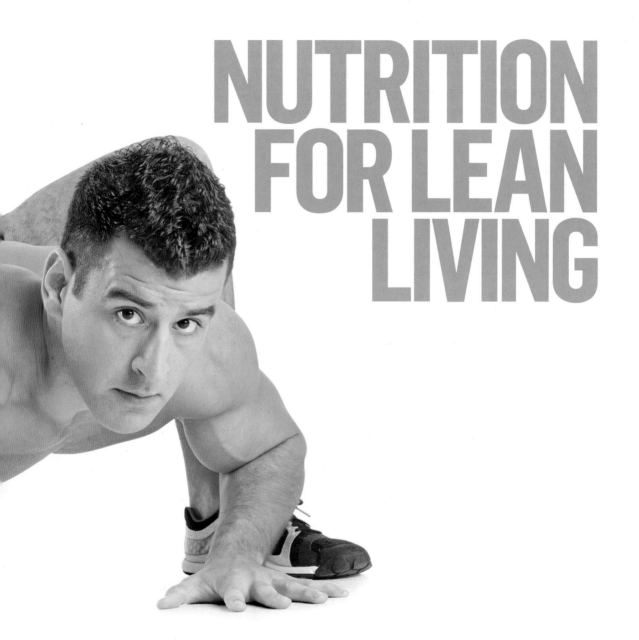

NUTRITION FOR LEAN LIVING

Eat to Incinerate Fat and Fuel Your Workouts

BY MICHAEL ROUSSELL, PhD

Mike Roussell holds a doctorate in nutrition from Pennsylvania State University. He is an author, a speaker, a weight-loss coach, and the founder of Naked Nutrition consulting. Dr. Roussell is also a nutritionist on *Men's Health* magazine's board of advisors.

A high-performance vehicle filled with regular gasoline will hesitate and sputter and won't deliver the high performance you expect when you step on the gas. Your body is similar. You need to fuel it right to make it work optimally. That's even more critical when you are making the kind of demands of it that you find in the extreme bodyweight exercise programs in this book. To reap all the benefits of BJ's metabolism-scorching workouts, you need to create the proper metabolic environment that allows your body to access stored body fat and rebuild muscle bigger and stronger, while also providing the nutrients it needs for lifelong health.

You might expect that the nutrition prescription to achieve all this would be complicated and full of overly detailed caloric calculations—but it isn't! It's actually quite simple. There are just eight keys that'll give your body its best fighting chance to shed fat and develop a lean and muscular physique.

KEY 1 Eat Four Times per Day

The first thing I want you to do is eat more often. Don't worry about calories right now. It's more important to establish the habit before you start fine-tuning. Let your hunger level determine how much you eat. To illustrate this for clients, I use a rule called Eat and Eat Again.

"You can eat as much as you want at any given meal, but you need to be able to eat that exact same amount of food 2 to 3 hours later."

The rule works because it curbs how much you consume at any one meal. For example, devouring an entire pizza may seem like a good idea at 2:00 p.m. on the day you skipped breakfast and forgot to have lunch. But what if you knew you had to eat another entire pizza just 2 to 3 hours later? Not quite as appealing, is it? Following the Eat and Eat Again rule will curb your calorie intake automatically, without requiring much thought. Eating more frequently keeps cravings at bay by avoiding the swings from high to low blood sugar that cause cravings.

ACTION STEP: The best way to start is ensuring that you have breakfast, lunch, and dinner. What to eat? Take your cues from "Eight Power Foods" on page 17. Once you have that down, just add in a midmorning or midafternoon protein-rich snack. On the days you work out, replace that snack with your workout nutrition.

KEY 2 Limit Consumption of Sugars and Processed Foods

If I could have you make just one change to your diet with the greatest potential to impact your weight and health, this would be it. Foods are processed to increase their shelf life and improve taste. To accomplish those goals, the manufacturers remove nutrients and replace them with less-expensive, longer-lasting fillers. Refined flours and sugars are cheap, easy

fillers to use. But in exchange for cheap, tasty, and convenient food, you end up with weight gain and worsened health. Nutrition research consistently shows that people who eat the most vegetables and fresh fruit have the best health outcomes, while those who consume the most processed food have the highest risk for heart disease, obesity, certain cancers, diabetes, and even premature death. The goal of Key 2 is to get you away from the things that make you fat and unhealthy.

Dietary displacement is the key to making this work. What you *don't* eat is just as important as what you do. A diet that's loaded with highly processed food prevents you from eating fruit, vegetables, and lean protein. Conversely, when you make the move from bar codes to bags, a diet rich in fruits and vegetables (foods that you have to put into bags) means eating less of the refined convenience food (things that come in boxes and packages with bar codes).

ACTION STEP: It's a two-part strategy: Start by identifying processed and sugar-sweetened foods that you are currently eating. Then make a list of fresh, or at least minimally processed, foods to replace them. For example, instead of grabbing yogurt with fruit on the bottom (that fruit comes with added sugars), choose plain yogurt with fresh berries. Putting Key 2 into action isn't easy, but it's the most important adjustment you can make.

KEY 3 Eat Fresh Stuff throughout the Day

As a world-renowned expert in obesity and eating behavior, Barbara Rolls, PhD, of Pennsylvania State University has shown repeatedly in her research that the *energy density* of your food is the single most important predictor of how many total calories you'll consume. An example of an energy-dense food is a bowl of pasta with a cream-based sauce: high density, low volume, tons of calories. By contrast, vegetables, because of their high fiber and water content, offer a high volume of food that can fill your plate and your stomach yet provide a low-calorie punch. Including them reduces the energy density of your meal, meaning you can eat a lot of vegetables at one sitting but still end up with a very low-calorie meal.

ACTION STEP: Only 6 percent of us meet the recommended daily minimums for fruit and vegetable consumption. The average American eats just over 1 cup of fruit and $\frac{1}{2}$ cup of vegetables each day. Make a deal with yourself: Every time you eat, have a piece of fruit or a vegetable; it is even better if you make them the foundation of your plate. If you've put Key 2 into action, then you should already have a lot more fresh fruits and vegetables around your house to include.

KEY 4 Drink More Water and Eliminate Calorie-Containing Beverages

Just about everyone can benefit from drinking more water. By properly hydrating your body, you'll be less fatigued and more alert, perform better, think straighter, and just feel better in general. Water is the very best performance-enhancing substance there is. A proper level of hydration before, during, and after exercise has been shown to help maintain performance, lower exercise heart rate, and reduce heat stress.

Many of us take in plenty of fluids, but we do it in the worst possible way. If you currently drink nondiet soda, lattes (or any other coffee-type drink that costs more than $5), or fruit juice throughout the day, you should stop. Replacing these calorie-containing drinks with water and/or unsweetened tea (especially green tea, which is high in antioxidants and has been shown to elevate fat burn) will make a huge difference in your health and body composition. If you drink two 20-ounce bottles of Coke or Pepsi each day, that's an extra 500 calories in your diet from which you get no nutritional benefit whatsoever. Think of it as a direct deposit into your lower abdomen. But by simply replacing those two sodas each day with water or another calorie-free beverage, you could lose a pound a week initially. Remember: *Drinking empty calories is wasting calories.*

ACTION STEP: This is the easiest key to put into action. Just stop drinking calories! The major sources are coffee drinks with added sugar and/or cream (not the packet of sugar in your coffee but the 400-calorie Frappuccino-type drinks), soda, sweetened or flavored water (such as Vitaminwater), sports drinks, and fruit juice. I'm not asking you to cut out sugar-sweetened beverages cold turkey. For starters, switch from Coke to Coke Zero, Gatorade to low-calorie Gatorade, and sweetened iced tea to artificially sweetened tea. Once you've made and adjusted to those switches, start replacing them with water or unsweetened tea.

KEY 5 Consume Lean Protein throughout the Day

Eating protein every time you have a meal is a strategy that is misunderstood by most involved in health and fitness. Bodybuilders will have you constantly eating boatloads of protein, while many dietitians and health professionals warn against high protein by using scare tactics born out of misinterpretation of scientific literature.

How much protein do you need? "Need" is an interesting concept. It sounds concrete, but what kind of need are we describing? To survive? To prevent a protein deficiency? To lose weight? To perform as an athlete at an elite level? To maximize the results of training? To live a long, active life?

The US Department of Agriculture has an RDA, or Recommended Dietary Allowance, for all nutrients, including protein. Here's how RDA is defined: *the average daily dietary nutrient intake level sufficient to meet the nutrient requirement of nearly all (97 to 98 percent) healthy individuals in a particular life stage and gender group.*

The RDA for protein for the average man is 60 to 65 grams per day. So if you eat 60 grams of protein a day—the equivalent of a 12-ounce sirloin steak or a couple chicken breasts—you won't die from not having enough protein (97 to 98 percent of the time). Essential amino acid deficiency is rarely an issue, so I'm less concerned about that and more interested in what the *optimal protein* intake is to help you reach your goals the fastest. When it comes to building muscle and losing fat, research consistently shows that doubling the RDA spaced out throughout the day is the path you want to take to get the best results the fastest.

PROTEIN TIMING AND PROTEIN SYNTHESIS

Our traditional view of protein has proved to be rather archaic. In addition to focusing on eating the minimum amount of protein required to prevent deficiencies, we have paid little attention to *how* we go about getting protein in our diet. Most Americans eat a large portion of protein at dinner, with smaller amounts of protein (if any) at breakfast and lunch. As you probably know, protein, and the amino acids that make it up, is required for building muscle. Your body, however, doesn't just use amino acids as the building blocks to construct your muscle. Your body uses amino acids to signal

EXERCISE AND CARBS
A MATCH MADE IN HEAVEN

After exercise, your muscles are in an energetic void, and they want nothing more than to restock their supplies. Your muscles store energy primarily as carbohydrates in the form of glycogen. Starches and simple sugars are key components for filling this void because of their fast-acting capabilities. At other times of the day, fast-acting carbohydrates can trigger excessive insulin release, which could favor the storage of carbohydrates in fat cells. Following exercise, however, fat storage isn't a priority for your body, and your muscle cells are primed to take in the carbohydrates that you eat. This is one of the few times that carbohydrates are preferentially shuttled to your muscle and away from cells. It is the perfect scenario for eating a carb-rich meal or snack. Unfortunately, we're accustomed to having sandwiches at lunch and building our dinners around starchy carbs like pasta and rice. When your goal is weight loss, a bread-heavy sandwich only works if it follows a midday workout. A pasta- or rice-based dinner is only a good idea on the days when you work out directly before you eat it. Most of us work out three or four times a week, and sometimes it can be difficult to adjust our meal plans to accommodate our postworkout needs. Soon enough, though, you'll plan to have carbs after workouts and establish a "new normal" eating pattern. And you'll get more pleasure from cinching your belt two notches tighter than you ever got from your lunchtime hoagie.

that it's time to *start up* the muscle-building machinery. The most important is an amino acid called leucine, which is found in just about every protein-containing food you eat.

For leucine to flip on the muscle-building switch, there needs to be a certain amount of protein present; this *protein threshold* must be reached to maximize protein synthesis. Scientists estimate that this threshold is about 30 grams of protein. Eat much more than 30 grams and you don't get extra protein synthesis. Now we can begin to see the tragic flaw of eating a steak dinner while ignoring protein earlier. Research from the University of Texas Medical Branch–Galveston shows us that by spreading our protein intake throughout the day (30 grams at breakfast, lunch, and dinner versus 90 grams at dinner), we end up with 25 percent more protein synthesis.

ACTION STEP: Eating more protein at lunch and dinner is easy for most of us. The tricky part is finding protein-rich snacks and breakfast ideas. For breakfast, go with eggs, lean breakfast meats, Greek yogurt, and smoothies with protein powder. For snacks, good options are Greek yogurt, nuts and seeds, roasted edamame beans, protein bars (with at least 10 grams of protein and no more than 30 grams of carbs), and protein shakes.

KEY 6 Use Starchy Foods for Postworkout Meals

Key 6 harnesses the power of what scientists call nutrient timing, which is the concept that certain foods benefit your body more at specific times of the day than at others. This makes innate sense to many of us. Others struggle with the idea, especially those folks who are still stuck on the idea that a calorie is a calorie. That old mantra about calories just isn't the case, especially during and after exercise. After exercise, your muscles want carbohydrates. This is why we want to preferentially eat starch-containing foods, or foods with a higher

density of carbohydrates, after workouts. What foods are in the starch category? Foods like rice, bread, pasta, oatmeal, cereal grains, quinoa, barley, corn, potatoes, and yams.

After exercise, your muscles are in an energy void, and they want nothing more than to restock their supply of carbohydrates in the form of glycogen. Starches and simple sugars are key components for filling this void because of their fast-acting capabilities. At most times of the day, an influx of fast-absorbing carbs will trigger excessive insulin release, which could favor the storage of carbohydrates in fat cells. Following exercise, however, your muscle cells are primed to take in the carbohydrates that you eat. This is one of the few times that carbs are preferentially shuttled to your muscle and away from fat cells. It is the perfect scenario.

ACTION STEP: Break the cultural habit of having sandwiches at lunch and building dinners around starchy carbs like pasta and rice. Plan to eat most of your fast-absorbing carbs soon after your workouts, and focus on proteins and high-fiber vegetables during other mealtimes.

KEY 7 Fuel Your Workouts

We talked about nutrient timing in our discussion of Keys 5 and 6. Now it is time to wrap up our discussion of nutrient timing with workout nutrition, the ultimate execution of nutrient timing. Exercise is a biochemical symphony involving the liberation of stored fat, the ridding of fatigue-signaling molecules from our muscles, and the breaking down of muscle so that it can be rebuilt stronger and more resilient for the next training session.

Properly executed workout nutrition can allow you to work harder for longer while also accelerating your recovery so that you come back bigger and stronger sooner. To accomplish this efficiently, we will segment workout nutrition into two phases. Phase 1 is performance and Phase 2 is recovery. Phase 1 occurs before

EIGHT POWER FOODS

Make sure these nutrition-packed ingredients show up in your regular meal rotation.

KEFIR

This cross between milk and yogurt is an excellent multipurpose food. Not only does kefir contain almost a 1:1 ratio of protein to carbohydrates, it also is an excellent source of healthy bacteria for your gut. These bacteria improve digestion and boost immune function.

TEA

The combination of caffeine and antioxidants found in green tea is famous for its fat-burning effects. Plus, research in the *American Journal of Clinical Nutrition* shows that a unique amino acid in tea called theanine can work in concert with caffeine to enhance focus, creativity, and your ability to multitask.

LEAN BEEF

Beef is known for its protein, but almost 50 percent of the fat in beef is the coveted monounsaturated fat. Unlike poultry, lean beef is a gold mine of nutrients: zinc, vitamin B_{12}, selenium, phosphorus, iron, vitamin B_6, and niacin. The leanest cuts are those described as loin or roast.

SPROUTED GRAIN BREAD

Bread is never considered a power food, but sprouted grain bread is the exception. The sprouting process makes many of the grain's nutrients more accessible to your body and converts some of the carbohydrates to protein. Sprouted grain bread products are a minimally processed, high-fiber way to get your bread fix and feel good about it.

ALMONDS

A unifying habit of lean and healthy people is that they snack on nuts. Almonds have a unique nutrient package, containing fiber, magnesium, and a truckload of vitamin E. Don't shy away from nuts due to their high fat content. Research from Purdue University shows that snacking on $1\frac{1}{2}$ ounces of almonds each day decreases hunger.

EXTRA VIRGIN OLIVE OIL

This oil is more than just high in monounsaturated fat. It contains high levels of powerful antioxidants called polyphenols. These polyphenols are considered by some scientists to be one of the main reasons why the Mediterranean diet is so heart healthy. To get the maximum antioxidant punch from your olive oil, look for first-pressed extra virgin olive oil sold in a dark glass bottle, and never cook with it at high temperatures.

BROCCOLI

Broccoli is a nutritional powerhouse of low-impact carbohydrates, fiber, and anticancer and anti-estrogen antioxidants. Three cups of raw broccoli contain fewer than 100 calories but are still satiating when eaten raw, sautéed, or roasted. Just never boil it, as this leaches out the nutrients. Also, pass on frozen broccoli. Research from the University of Illinois shows that the blanching process used on broccoli before it is frozen prevents the activation of some of broccoli's anticancer antioxidants.

EGGS

Initially banished to the "do not eat" list due to their cholesterol content, eggs are now a "must eat" food. Recent research shows very little relationship between the cholesterol you eat and the levels of cholesterol in your blood. Eggs are the gold standard for high-quality protein and amino acids. Plus, the yolks are also rich in choline, which is a key nutrient for brain function.

and during your workouts, while Phase 2 occurs immediately after your workout ends.

PHASE 1—PERFORMANCE: Never work out in a fasted state. The small increased potential of burning more calories from fat while training fasted is outweighed by the greater intensity with which you will be able to perform if you have properly fueled. For BJ's short, intense workouts, you don't need to consume carbohydrate drinks and gels as if you were running a marathon. Instead, you only need to have eaten within the last 2 hours. This will ensure that your blood sugar levels are primed to fuel an intense workout, but the meal is far enough away from your training session that you won't "lose it" while training. If you are

EIGHT KEY SUPPLEMENTS

FISH OIL

These concentrated long-chain omega-3 fatty acids impact multiple areas of your body, from improving heart health and joint function to hindering fat cell growth. What to do: Take 1 to 2 grams of EPA and DHA per day with a meal.

CAFFEINE

The source of your morning coffee's power is also a highly researched performance booster with benefits ranging from increased endurance and improved reaction time to decreased perception of muscle pain during exercise. You can get a boost from the caffeine in your coffee, but the caffeine levels in coffee are very variable. What to do: Pop 200 milligrams of caffeine in tablet form and increase the dose based on your individual tolerance. It takes around 45 minutes for caffeine levels to peak in your blood, so plan accordingly based on when you are going to exercise.

VITAMIN D

This vitamin actually acts more like a hormone. Vitamin D is needed for proper bone and immune health. Low levels of vitamin D have been associated with obesity and poor blood sugar control. What to do: Take 2,000 IU per day with a meal. Have your doctor run a vitamin D blood test to further optimize your daily dose.

MAGNESIUM

This mineral is generally underdosed in multivitamins. It is needed for more than 300 reactions in the body, and it promotes relaxation. What to do: Take 400 milligrams of chelated magnesium before bed.

CREATINE

It's one of the most-vetted sports supplements on the market. In addition to making you more powerful, creatine impacts brain function and helps you get better results with your training during periods of high stress. What to do: Take 5 grams of creatine monohydrate in your carbohydrate-based preworkout performance shake.

MULTIVITAMIN

This is the cheapest nutritional insurance policy you can take out on your body to ensure that it has all the vitamin and mineral cofactors it needs. What to do: Take one multivitamin per day with a meal.

WHEY PROTEIN POWDER

This king of protein powders is not just loaded with muscle-building leucine but is also rapidly digested, giving your body key amino acids fast when it needs them. What to do: Have a protein shake containing 20 to 30 grams of whey protein directly after exercise.

ZINC

Intense exercise can deplete this key mineral, yielding decreases in thyroid function and testosterone. What to do: Take 30 milligrams of zinc anytime during the day.

training first thing in the morning, then drinking 16 to 20 ounces of a sports beverage shortly after waking will be sufficient to prime your body, due to the drink's ability to accelerate digestion.

PHASE 2—RECOVERY: The combination of strategic nutrition and exercise offers the unique opportunity to boost your body's muscle-building capacity by 100 percent followed by an additional and sustained increase for the next 24 to 36 hours. Here's why: Right after exercise, your body switches from performance mode to recovery mode. We need to address your body's recovery needs in two different ways: refilling drained energy stores and rebuilding broken-down muscle. In Key 6 we talked about corralling carbohydrate-dense foods (breads, pastas, etc.) into the several hours following exercise. In addition to your muscles having a greater affinity for carbohydrates during this time, they are more adept at refilling their glycogen/sugar stores (which you use during your training sessions). This is another reason why it is a good idea to have carbohydrate-dense foods following exercise.

When you finish your workout and your body switches over to recovery mode, it starts rebuilding muscle so that it can come back stronger and bigger for your next training session. Research shows that the act of exercise itself increases protein synthesis. You can supercharge the effect by consuming protein right after you exercise. Leading muscle protein synthesis researchers say it is important to wait until *after* you have finished exercise to have protein so that the amino acid spike in your bloodstream matches up with your body's exercise-induced increase in protein synthesis. It is a perfect storm of muscle building.

ACTION STEPS: To enhance your performance during BJ's short, intense workouts, ensure that you have eaten within the last $1\frac{1}{2}$ to 2 hours *but no less than $\frac{1}{2}$ hour before your workout.* Your blood sugar levels will be primed

to fuel an intense workout, but you won't feel full while training. To enhance recovery, have 20 to 30 grams of whey protein right after exercise. That will add gasoline to the protein-synthesis fire sparked by your training session. Whey protein is a rapidly digested protein source loaded with leucine that will help maximize protein synthesis quickly. Then, within 2 hours of your training, have a solid food meal that contains carbohydrate-dense foods like breads, grains, or pasta.

KEY 8 Rely on Habits, Not Brute Force Willpower

Research regarding the power of the human will and self-control yields remarkable findings about how much we can accomplish through sheer willpower alone. However, our willpower reserves are still finite and readily depleted by stress, distraction, and concentrated effort in other areas of life. This is why *willing* yourself to stick to your diet is a short-sighted strategy that rarely leads to long-term leanness and weight-loss success.

Dietary approaches that yield long-term success are those that allow you to never have to lose the same 10 pounds a second (or third!) time. These approaches are rooted in habit, like the habit of brushing your teeth. You never have to think about brushing; you just do it. Imagine if healthy eating was like that. Well, you *can* make the seven previous nutrition keys nearly automatic.

ACTION STEPS: Focus on one or two of the keys in this chapter at a time. For example, put all your effort into eating protein at each meal, nothing else. Spend 2 to 3 weeks drilling that into your daily routine. Once protein-rich meals and snacks become second nature, then it is time to move to another key, like cutting out sugar-sweetened drinks. Continue this methodical approach to nutrition habit mastery and you will be amazed at how a once-daunting concept like fat loss becomes easy.

Chapter 3

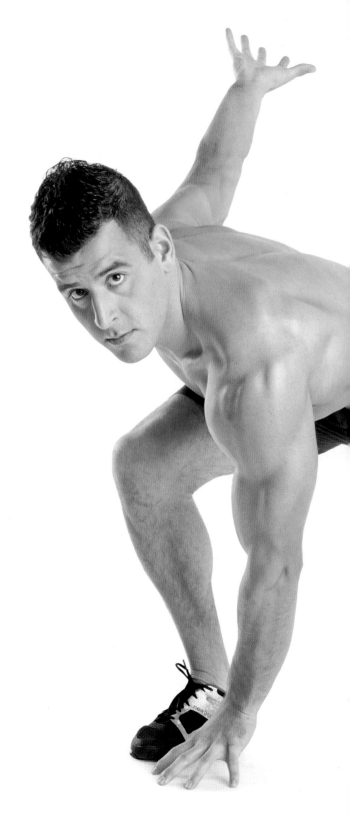

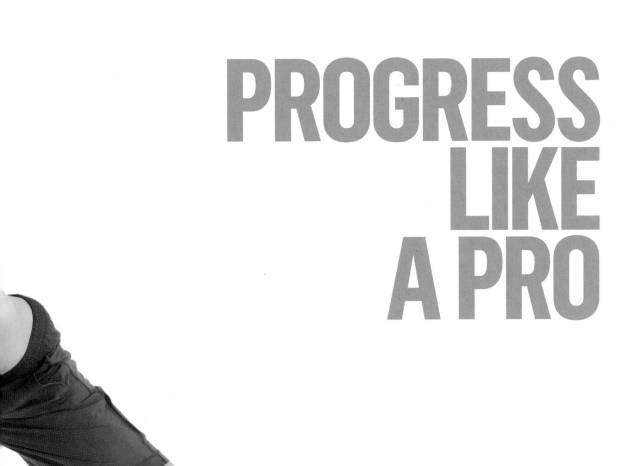

PROGRESS LIKE A PRO

As simple, useful, and beneficial as bodyweight training is, there's one aspect that makes it a little more challenging to use than, say, free-weight training: It doesn't have a quantifiable way to measure your progress. With weights, it's super easy to track success: If you increase the weight you're lifting, you're getting stronger. Plus, you can add weight in 2.5- to 45-pound increments to provide the needed progressive overload to make a change.

No training system or tool is perfect, but there's a way to fix this shortcoming in bodyweight training: with a system of intelligent progressions. My goal in this chapter is to empower you with the ability to make any bodyweight exercise harder or easier instantly. There are dozens of ways to take any bodyweight movement and make it feel 5 to 10 pounds heavier or lighter just like with weights.

These progressions and regressions can be accomplished through simple tweaks to your body position or by using everyday items like chairs, benches, boxes, towels, poles, ropes, tree branches, walls, water jugs, broomsticks, heavy rocks, etc., or by using commercial fitness tools such as dumbbells, kettlebells, sandbags, resistance bands, weight vests, weight plates, chinup bars, suspension trainers like the TRX, and more. The point is that you can make the exercises harder by adding mechanical resistance or you can do it totally equipment free. The options are really endless, which is why bodyweight training is so versatile and useful for virtually anyone of any fitness level who wants to improve his or her body and strength. Let's review how to use these tools and methods to scale any exercise.

IT'S ALL ABOUT LEVERAGE

Leverage is a mechanical advantage (or disadvantage) achieved through using a lever (or levers). In terms of your musculoskeletal system, your bones are the levers, your joints are the fulcrums, and your muscles are the movers that apply force. The less the mechanical advantage, the more muscular force that is required to create movement or to maintain certain positions. This forces your body to adapt by becoming stronger and more muscular. You can achieve a mechanical disadvantage (i.e., make a movement more difficult) by either:

- Changing your body position
- Lengthening or shortening the primary muscles involved beyond their natural, resting length

Force equals force. When it comes to progression, it doesn't matter how exactly you go about creating more muscular force, it just matters that you do. Though traditionally, increased force has been accomplished through lifting heavier weights, a mechanical disadvantage can make your muscles work harder, or create more force, which makes the exercise feel "heavier" without actually adding weight to the movement. Confused? Don't be. I'm going to break all of this down for you step-by-step so you can maximize every rep to the fullest.

THE SEVEN WAYS TO SCALE ANY EXERCISE

Here are your options for making any exercise harder or easier. Note that when you scale certain dynamic exercises, you may use several different types of scaling. For example, moving from a Split Squat to a Forward Lunge technically employs progressions in stability, tempo, and complexity.

1 External Loading

This is the most basic progression there is: Increase the load to make an exercise harder or decrease the load to make an exercise easier. You can add an external load with weight plates, barbells, dumbbells, kettlebells, medicine balls, sandbags, chains, and resistance bands, or even outdoor implements like rocks or logs. In terms of bodyweight training, some examples include:

- Holding on to any of these implements to make lower-body exercises like Squats, Lunges, and Stepups more difficult
- Placing these implements on your lap to make glute exercises like Hip Thrusts and back exercises like Rows more challenging or putting them on your back to make core exercises like Pushups and Planks more intense
- Hanging weights on or around your trunk or shoulders to make Hangs or Pullups harder

One of my favorite ways to add an external load is using a weight vest. It's less cumbersome and more natural, and it provides for easier setups and transitions. A good weight vest fits snugly to your trunk so it doesn't move around on you during training. It also shouldn't impede the natural movement of your arms, shoulders, or hips. I like adjustable weight vests that allow you to quickly increase or decrease the load. My favorite weight vests are produced by Hyperwear.

Other than weight vests, resistance bands are the safest, easiest, and most convenient way to add an external load to most bodyweight movements. Resistance bands provide a dynamic variable resistance that peaks toward the top of a movement and tends to be easier on your joints than dead weight. You can wrap a band around your trunk and hold the ends with your hands to make Pushups and Planks harder or place it around your hips with your hands pressed into the floor to make Hip Thrusts more difficult. You can secure one end of the band to your feet and attach the other end to your shoulders or hands to make Squat variations tougher. Another option is to anchor a band to the floor and wrap it around your shoulders to make Pullups a beastly task. Or to assist you on Pullups, anchor the band to the Pullup bar and secure the other end to your body. I recommend the continually looped and color-coded elastic bands that you can find at resistancebandtraining.com.

You can also unload your body weight with self-assisted squatting exercises by placing your hands on any stable support system like a pole, railing, or door frame or by holding on to the handles of a suspension training system like a TRX. This is a particularly useful rehab technique for those with a history of lower-body injuries. It's also a great tool for active recovery between workouts or for higher-rep endurance training.

2 Relative Loading

Relative loading refers to the use of leverage to shift more weight onto the working muscles and joints involved in a given movement. This can be accomplished by changing your body angle or your joint angle.

Body angle describes the relationship between your body and the floor. There's no better exercise to demonstrate body-angle progressions than the Pushup. Beginners start performing Pushups with the hands elevated on a bench, wall, or table, because this position shifts the weight from the upper to lower body, making the exercise easier. From there, you progressively decrease the elevation until you can finally perform the classic Pushup with your hands on the floor and your body parallel to the ground. Researchers at the University of Athens found that the standard floor Pushup forces your upper body to lift 66 percent of your body weight, so that gives you a little gauge regarding the relative load with easier inclined versions. Technically, at an incline of 45 degrees, you should be lifting about 33 percent of your body weight. We progress the exercise by elevating your feet to shift more of your weight onto your hands to make the exercise harder. The master step is being able to perform a Handstand Pushup with your body completely inverted so that you are pressing 100 percent of your body weight.

Joint angle describes the position of your primary joints during a given exercise. Using the Pushup again, a classic floor Pushup is performed with your hands directly underneath your shoulders. Here your shoulders are flexed at 90 degrees, and you have the biggest mechanical advantage because you can fully move both your elbow and shoulder joints and use your triceps, pecs, and shoulders to create force. This is an example of a bent-limb exercise. But if you use a high hand placement by moving your arms more in front of your body until they are eventually fully extended overhead, without changing your body angle, you make the Pushup a lot harder to perform. This is because your elbow joints can't produce as much torque and your triceps can't assist as much in the movement. Thus, your shoulders have to do most of the work. This same thing happens when you abduct your shoulders 90 degrees to each side, in what I call an Iron Cross Pushup. With the elbows locked in extension, the triceps can't assist in the movement, and now the chest muscles are working overtime. Both the overhead Pushup and the Iron Cross are examples of straight-limb exercises. Straight-limb movements are significantly harder to perform than bent-limb movements because movement is limited at one or more joints. Plus, the primary muscles involved are either shortened or stretched beyond their natural resting length, making it more difficult for them to produce force to execute the movement.

3 Stability

Stability describes that constant interaction between your center of gravity and your body's base of support. Using stability progressions instead of loading progressions will make your movements more functional and athletic, recruit more of your core and balancing muscles, and better stabilize your joints. It's really just a smarter way to exercise.

Outlined following is the full spectrum of stability progressions.

A. BASE OF SUPPORT

The wider your base of support, the more stable you are and the less distance you need to travel to execute a movement. The narrower your base of support, the less stable you are and the greater distance you need to travel to execute the movement. Think of a Pushup with your hands close together, thumbs touching. Narrower bases make exercise more challenging; a wide base of support, with your center of mass positioned within that base, makes exercises easier to perform because you're most stable and the range of motion of the exercise is automatically decreased.

B. CENTER OF GRAVITY

Though we all have different body dimensions and varied trunk and limb lengths, for our purposes, let's just say that your belly button is your center of mass when in a normal standing position with your arms at your sides. This basically cuts your body in half.

Now, your center of gravity can be adjusted either vertically or horizontally to make an exercise harder or easier. For example, extending your arms more overhead with a more upright torso makes a bodyweight Squat harder to perform. Horizontal adjustments include moving your center of gravity closer to the axis of rotation (the moving or stabilizing joints) to make the Squat easier or moving your center of gravity farther away to make it harder. Using the Squat again, if you hold a heavy weight on your shoulders at chest level, it's an easier Squat than holding that same weight with your arms fully extended in front of your body. That's because the load is positioned farther from the axes of rotation (in this case, your hips, knees, and ankles) and your base of support (feet).

C. POINTS OF CONTACT

The more points of contact, the more stable you are and the easier the exercise is to perform. The fewer the points of contact, the less stable you are and the harder the exercise is to per-

form. This is why Single-Arm Pushups are harder than two-arm Pushups, why Single-Leg Squats are harder than two-leg Squats, and why planking on one arm, one leg, or one arm and one leg is harder than planking on both hands and feet.

It's also important to note how much total surface area of your body is in contact with the floor. For example, doing Pushups with your hands flat on the floor is more stable than doing them on your fists because less total surface area is supported by the fists. Doing a Pushup on your fingertips is even harder (even though it's 10 points of contact versus 2 in the previous examples) because you have the least amount of surface-area contact with a stable surface. It's the same thing with squatting on your toes versus squatting with your feet flat on the floor—Toe Squats are much harder because you're less stable.

This concept of surface area also applies to what I call "tweener" exercises in between two-limb and one-limb movements. In the case of Squats, Staggered or Split Squats have you squatting with one foot flat on the floor while on the toes of the other foot. In the case of Pushups, uneven or Archer Pushups have you pushing with one hand flat on the floor while on the fingertips of the other hand. In both cases, the exercises are harder than the two-limb version but easier than the one-limb version, making them key stepping-stone exercises to the advanced movements within their respective categories.

D. STATIC VERSUS DYNAMIC BASE OF SUPPORT CONTACT

An exercise is most stable when your points of contact with the ground remain connected throughout the duration of the movement. However, when you remove this connection at any time during the movement, it increases the stability demands and makes the exercise harder. For example, let's compare a Split Squat with a Lunge. Technically, it's a similar movement pattern, as the bottom of each move is identical in both exercises. However, with a Split Squat, both feet remain in contact with the ground from start to finish, whereas with a Lunge, you are either stepping forward (or backward) to get into the bottom of the Split Squat position. A Split Squat provides a static base of support for the full duration of the exercise. A Lunge provides a dynamic base of support, where you move from a position of high stability to a position of lower stability. That's why a Lunge is harder than a Split Squat. And anytime your feet leave the ground, the exercise becomes more challenging.

E. ASYMMETRICAL LOADING

An asymmetrical or uneven load is created when one side of your body has more weight on it than the other side. This creates tipping and rotation forces that require much greater midline stabilization. That's right, those delicious abdominal muscles need to step up their game!

For example, with a Single-Leg Hip Hinge, you can perform the exercise in an asymmetrical manner by reaching with one arm at a time or by having one hand closer to your center of mass and one hand farther away from your center of mass. The weight of your reaching arm creates uneven loading that requires your body to fight rotational forces, making the exercise harder to stabilize.

F. UNSTABLE SURFACE

Performing an exercise on a stable, even surface like the flat ground is easier than performing that same movement on an unstable, uneven surface like a pillow, Airex balance pad, or balance board. That's why running in sand is more difficult than running on pavement. That's also why performing Planks with your hands on a stability ball or with your feet in a suspension trainer is harder than performing that same Plank on the floor. A dynamic, fluid surface is more unstable and makes an exercise significantly more challenging.

4 Tempo

You can make an exercise harder by speeding up the movement or slowing it down. The tempo of an exercise includes four distinct components.

ECCENTRIC PERIOD (E): the time it takes to perform the negative or "lowering" portion of an exercise, when your muscles lengthen under tension. This is the deceleration phase of a movement, like hitting the brakes on your car. Your muscles are strongest during this portion of an exercise.

ECCENTRIC-CONCENTRIC TRANSITION PERIOD (EC): the time it takes to transition between the eccentric and concentric phase of an exercise, often called the midpoint of an exercise. Pausing at this position for any length of time creates an isometric muscular contraction where no movement at the joint(s) takes place.

CONCENTRIC PERIOD (C): the time it takes to perform the positive or "lifting" portion of an exercise, when your muscles shorten under tension. This is the acceleration phase of a movement, like hitting the gas and going pedal to metal when driving.

TRANSITION PERIOD BETWEEN REPETITIONS (T): the time you take between each repetition of an exercise.

For example, one way to make a traditional Pushup harder is to take 3 seconds to lower your chest to the floor (E), and then pause for 1 second as you reach the bottom of the Pushup without resting on the floor (EC), then explode back up to the starting position (C), and finally pause for 1 second before you perform the next repetition (T).

Before you try tempo progressions, be sure you've mastered a movement with perfect technique using 4 seconds to perform it at a controlled tempo of 2 seconds for lowering (E), 1-second pause (EC), explosive positive (C), and 1 second for transition (T). That's how you'll perform most of the basic moves in this book. When you are ready for tempo progression, try these.

GO FASTER TO BOOST POWER AND TRAINING DENSITY. Maximum power is trained by performing explosive work for bouts of 10 seconds or fewer or 5 reps or fewer. Power endurance is trained by performing explosive work for 20 seconds or longer or 10 reps or more. Power exercises are often known as plyometrics (or plyos). They take advantage of what's called the stretch-shortening cycle or stretch reflex, whereby a muscle rapidly lengthens and then quickly reverses its action. Examples include sprinting, jumping, hopping, leaping, bounding, etc. Power exercises also involve performing basic exercises like Pushups, Squats, and Lunges as fast as possible.

For example, if you want to build maximum power, you can perform sets of 3 to 5 Jump Squats with plenty of rest between sets, where you're trying to get as much height as you can on every rep. Using a harder Squat variation (such as a Split Jump Squat or Single-Leg Jump Squat) will result in slower velocities that develop more strength speed. Using an easier Squat variation (such as a regular Squat or Assisted Squat) will result in faster velocities that develop more speed strength. Both options are great and should be used for a well-rounded power-training program.

On the other side of the spectrum, you can build maximum endurance by performing as many Squats (or Jump Squats) as you can in, say, 30 seconds. It's obvious that performing 20 reps is a better result than 10 and means you've boosted your power output. This increase in reps can only be accomplished by performing the Squat at a faster speed than our 4-second tempo. Performing more work in the same amount of time increases training density (work performed per unit of time) and will help you burn more fat and build more lean muscle. However, increasing speed of movement is only a true progression when performed without sacrificing form or range of motion.

In addition, explosive tempos better target your powerful fast-twitch muscle fibers. These fibers are key to improving athleticism and reducing the risk of injury because they allow you to react quickly. These fibers are also the first to go with the age-related muscle loss that occurs in people over 30 years old, so you need to target fast-twitch muscles in your training. Plus, power training helps build powerful joints and connective tissues. But remember to always master an exercise at a slow speed before progressing to a faster speed or you risk overly stressing your joints.

GO SLOWER TO INCREASE MUSCLE WORK AND BULLETPROOF YOUR JOINTS. Your muscles and tendons are like coiled springs. When you perform the lowering/eccentric portion of any exercise, your muscles and tendons build up stored elastic energy that allows you to quickly uncoil or bounce back to the starting position. So when you sink your hips back quickly into a deep squatting position, the muscles of your lower body are primed to pop you right back up to the starting position just as a stretched rubber band would.

If you want your muscles to work harder, you need to avoid the bounce back of the released rubber band. You do that by using time. Studies show that it takes only 4 seconds to eliminate this stretch reflex and discharge all of the potential elastic energy within your muscles and tendons. The less elastic energy within your muscles, the harder your muscles must work and the less your joints and connective tissues must work to perform any exercise. The result is a greater total muscle fiber recruitment. For this reason, slowing a movement down is a great way to rehab an injury or bulletproof your joints.

One way to incorporate this 4-second time period into an exercise is to perform an isometric hold in the transition period between the eccentric and concentric portion. For example, perform a 4-second hold at the bottom position of a Pushup before returning to the starting position.

Another option is to take at least 4 seconds

before performing the concentric portion of the exercise. For example, in a Squat, you can take 3 seconds to lower your body into the bottom of the Squat and then pause for 1 second, which is a total of 4 seconds before you would actually push back up to the starting position.

One more thing to consider: Slow lowerings allow you to get used to more advanced exercise variations to bridge the gap between easier and harder moves. Simply perform the lowering portion only on advanced moves like Single-Leg Squats, Chinups, or Single-Arm Pushups. Once you can do multiple sets of multiple reps of slow eccentrics, you'll be in a great position to add the concentric phase and nail your first full-range-of-motion rep.

Finally, studies show that if you have the *intent* of performing the lifting or concentric portion on every rep of any given exercise as fast as humanly possible, you activate the most total muscle fibers. More muscles worked equals more calories burnt and greater gains in lean body mass.

GET STRONGER BY OWNING THE TOPS AND BOTTOMS. If you want to get better at an exercise, simply focus on improving your positioning at key points during an exercise. If you can own the top and the bottom of a given movement (or the start and midpoint, depending on the exercise), you'll own everything else in between. Apply this concept by focusing on isometric holds at the top and bottom of exercises like Pushups, Squats, and Pullups. This is especially useful for advanced moves that are currently beyond your reach, since your muscles are stronger eccentrically and isometrically than they are concentrically.

When it comes to iso holds, you're strongest at the starting position and weakest at the midpoint position. Don't just hold it; try to create as much total-body tension as possible for maximum benefits. At first, you might be able to muster only a couple seconds at a time, but gradually you'll build up this holding pattern until:

- You can comfortably hold the starting position of a move (the top of a Squat or Pushup and the bottom of a Pullup) for at least 60 seconds.

- You can comfortably hold the midpoint position of a move (the bottom of a Squat or Pushup and the top of a Pullup) for at least 30 seconds.

Once you can accomplish this, you should have no trouble crushing that movement.

5 Range of Motion (ROM)

Full range of motion is when you perform an exercise from the absolute top to the absolute bottom and back. However, ROM can be altered to make an exercise harder or easier.

EXTENDED ROM is when you perform an exercise through a greater total distance. This makes the same move harder without the need for external resistance or additional loading. For example, if you perform a Pushup with your hands supported on dumbbells, medicine balls, or low boxes that are placed on the floor, you allow your chest to lower farther than it normally would if your hands were placed on the floor.

Another example of an extended ROM progression includes performing a greater amount of work in the most difficult portion of a given exercise for every rep. For example, when performing a Pushup or Squat variation, first lower yourself to the bottom of the movement, then come back up only halfway, then go all the way down again before coming all the way up to the original starting position. This is called a 1.5 rep and has you performing twice as many repetitions during the bottom of the movement where it's most challenging.

BLOCKED ROM is when you perform an exercise with a different starting and/or end point than normal. For example, performing Pushups starting halfway down and only moving between there and the bottom position can be more challenging than a regular full ROM Pushup because you're keeping your chest muscles under constant tension without resting at the top of the movement as usual after each rep. This "constant tension" technique has been used by bodybuilders for decades to boost new muscle growth, particularly for lagging body parts.

Another way to block ROM is by breaking down a work set into two or three parts. In the case of a Pushup, a two-part block could have you perform a certain number of reps in the bottom half of a Pushup and then a certain number of reps in the top half of a Pushup within the same work set. A three-part block would be similar, except it would break the Pushup into the top third, mid-third, and bottom third. Blocking provides a new stimulus that can strengthen sticking points and spark new muscle growth.

PARTIAL ROM is a modified or shortened range of motion to make an exercise easier. Classic examples include Half Pushups, where you lower your body halfway down and back up, and a Half Pullup, where you pull your body halfway up and back down. This allows you to cheat to get more total reps and build confidence with harder exercise variations. It also can be a way to extend a set and perform more total work after no longer being able to complete full ROM reps. However, the goal is eventually to be able to perform these exercises through a full ROM on a regular basis.

6 Complexity

You can increase the complexity of an exercise and reward yourself with more benefits by:

A. COMBINING MULTIPLE JOINTS OR MUSCLES

Moving one joint—called an isolation or single-joint movement—is easier for your body to figure out than moving multiple joints at once—called a compound or multijoint move-ment. There's just less skill required in the former. For example, performing a Biceps Curl with dumbbells (a single-joint move) is easier to master than performing a Pullup, where your shoulders and core muscles are called into play. Though isolation exercises are often considered useless exercises for meathead bodybuilders, they do have their place in a sound training program, especially early on.

For example, being able to properly perform an isolated movement like a Pullup Shrug should be a prerequisite before anyone ever attempts a full Pullup. To perform a Pullup Shrug, start by holding on to a bar or a pair of rings from a Dead Hang, where your arms are fully extended overhead and your shoulder blades are fully protracted and elevated so that your shoulders rest by your ears. Now, moving only at the shoulder girdle and keeping your arms straight, pull your shoulders down and back and lift your chest up while keeping your ribs down and abs braced. This finishing position is how you should initiate every single Pullup rep you ever do for optimal shoulder health. Finally, reverse the movement and repeat for time or reps.

Even though this move is recommended for beginners, it's a great corrective exercise for advanced users because it activates the key pulling muscles of your lats and middle to lower traps, muscles that tend to turn off with poor posture and excessive pushing movements. It also requires excellent shoulder and thoracic spine mobility (and core stabilization) to get into a safe overhead position without hyperextending your lower back and shrugging your shoulders. This makes such a single-joint, isolation movement like a Pullup Shrug both a great beginner move and a great warmup drill before a multijoint compound movement like Pullups.

B. COMBINING MULTIPLE PLANES OF MOTION

The body moves in three basic planes of movement: *sagittal*—movements that occur front to back and up and down; *frontal*—movements that occur side to side; and *transverse*—rotational movements.

The vast majority of the exercises that most people perform occur mostly in the sagittal plane, such as Squats and Bench Presses (or Pushups). In other words, the frontal and transverse planes are highly neglected, creating a training imbalance that can lead to a host of unwanted short- and long-term injuries. It's critical to exercise in all three planes in a sound training program.

One way to accomplish this is to take a uniplanar exercise and make it multiplanar by combining it with one or more planes of movement. The more planes of movement you incorporate, the harder the exercise and the more muscles you work. The Lunge is a good exercise to illustrate this point.

❶ Sagittal plane Lunge variation: FORWARD LUNGE

❷ Frontal plane Lunge variation: LATERAL LUNGE

❸ Transverse plane Lunge variation: ROTATIONAL LUNGE

You can combine two or more of these Lunges to make one multiplane exercise.

Here's how you would combine all three: Step with your right foot into a Forward Lunge, then return to the starting position. Next, step with your right foot into a Lateral Lunge and return. Finally, step into a Rotational Lunge, then return to the starting position. Repeat for time, then do the same exercise while stepping with the left foot.

It's much more challenging for your nervous system to incorporate multiple planes of movement at once—in addition to the fact that more muscles are worked and more energy is expended.

C. COMBINING MULTIPLE MOVEMENT PATTERNS

Combination moves, like the triple Lunge we just discussed, are harder than individual exercises and should be treated that way. They require much greater skill and motor control.

Take as an example the Burpee, the ultimate equipment-free total-body exercise. It combines hinging, squatting, planking, pushing, and jumping movements into one seamless sweat maker. No other exercise works more muscles and burns more calories per minute than this big nasty, which is why *it sucks!* Perfect execution of this move is also a sign of elite athleticism and functional fitness.

The Burpee is probably the most bastardized exercise on the planet. That's because most people can't perform a perfect, full ROM Squat or Pushup to start (not to mention hip hinging, planking, and jumping). Dysfunction plus more dysfunction equals disaster and catastrophic bodily harm. If you want to master a complex combination skill like a Burpee, you should first master the easier individual components before progressing to that level of movement proficiency.

7 Metabolic Demand (or Stress)

This progression category makes an exercise harder to perform by increasing the metabolic demand on your body. There are three ways to do this.

A. CUT REST PERIODS

Your body needs at least 2 minutes and upwards of 10 minutes for complete recovery between sets of a given exercise. If you cut your rest periods down to 30 to 60 seconds, your muscles never fully recover, making the same exercise feel a lot harder.

There are pros and cons to any change in programming variables. In this case, the pros are that you make the same move harder without changing it in any way or adding an external load. The cons are that you will feel weaker and be unable to perform as many reps as you normally would under conditions of full recovery. In other words, you're building more endurance and less strength.

B. CHANGE EXERCISE ORDER

Another way to increase the metabolic stress on your body is to mix up your exercise order with alternating sets, where you perform multiple moves back-to-back. Alternating sets can be broken into two categories: competitive and noncompetitive.

Noncompetitive alternating sets pair two or more moves that work different muscle groups or movement patterns so as not to impair your recovery between exercises. Examples include alternating between upper-body and lower-body exercises like Pushups and Squats. This tactic is great for increasing fat loss, metabolic conditioning, and training density. Grouping exercises that work different areas of your body allows you to rest from one exercise while working another without actually needing to take time to rest.

Competitive alternating sets pair two or more moves that work similar muscle groups and movement patterns to increase the local muscular endurance demand and accumulate more muscle damage. For example, if I had you pair Squats with Lunges, by the time you got to the Lunges, your legs would already be fatigued. The same thing would happen if I paired Handstand Pushups with regular Pushups or Pullups with Rows. Because you're prefatiguing your working muscles, the subsequent exercise becomes much harder than if you just performed straight sets of single exercises with full rest.

C. INCREASE TRAINING VOLUME

Training volume describes the total number of sets and reps you do. It can be divided into two basic components: daily and weekly training volume.

For example, if you did 3 sets of 10 Squats, that's 30 total Squat reps in that single training session. Or you could commit to doing 30 reps of Squats per day each week (that's 210 total reps over the course of a week). Both options describe daily training volume.

Now, weekly training volume describes the total number of sets and reps you do for a given exercise within a single week of training. Using the example above, if you did the 3 sets of 10-rep Squat workout three times per week, that would result in 90 total Squats that week. But if you opted for the 30 reps of Squats per day alternative, that would translate into a larger weekly training volume of 210 reps on the Squat. Clearly, the second option is harder.

So increasing your daily or weekly training volume with a given exercise is a final way to make the same exercise harder without adding weight. Gradually progressing to 40 Squats a day, then to 50 and so forth, is a guaranteed way to build more muscle and improve your fitness. However, the drawbacks with endless increases in volume are excessive muscle soreness and larger time requirements. That's why I recommend you typically keep your per-workout training volume for a given move to about 25 to 50 reps, which is what many fitness experts agree to be the sweet spot for building muscle, improving strength, and boosting metabolism. Instead of adding more volume, intensify the exercise by using one of the endless progression options above.

4

Chapter

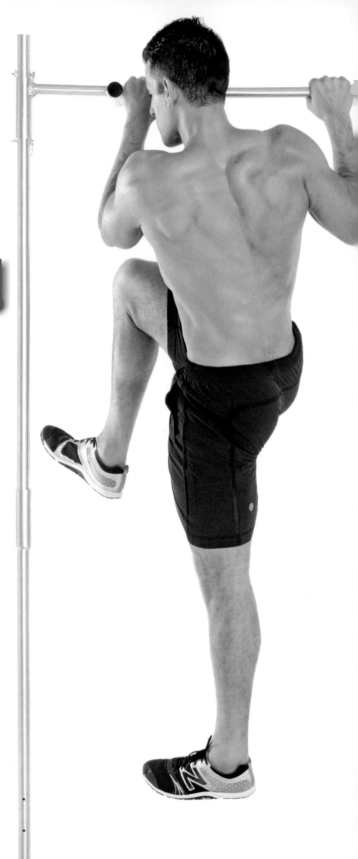

THE BODYWEIGHT 8 EXERCISES

Welcome to the foundation of a fit body, what I call the Bodyweight 8 exercises. They are the eight bodyweight exercises that you will be using religiously to get into the best shape of your life. Over the course of the following chapters, you will learn everything you'll ever need to know about these movements, including:

- The benefits of each exercise
- How to master each move with flawless form
- The step-by-step progressions to take you from ground zero to superhero
- The top variations for each exercise

Before we start learning them, it's important to understand the philosophy behind this selection of movements. And I want to teach you some global concepts that you will use throughout the book. Get ready to become the master of the universe that is your body.

MASTER FEWER MOVES

Next to lack of motivation, the biggest roadblock for most people who start a fitness program is a condition I call "exercise attention deficit disorder," or "workout ADD." Most people treat exercises like flavors at their favorite ice-cream shop, endlessly mixing and matching exercises or switching to completely different workouts from week to week or month to month out of boredom or lack of focus. Though this approach may be pleasing to your palate when it comes to ice cream, it will most certainly leave you with a bad taste in your mouth when it comes to exercise.

Consistency is the most important factor for long-term success with a fitness routine. It takes your body and brain a good amount of time to figure out how to most efficiently perform a movement. When you constantly switch things up, you'll never be able to fully master the various skills associated with perfectly executing an exercise. *But what about the idea of constantly challenging muscles with new moves?* you may be asking. *Isn't that the way to spur growth?* While it's true that shocking your muscles out of a long routine has benefits to the longtime exerciser, I firmly believe that most people, especially beginners, are better off sticking to fewer exercises and milking every last bit of benefit out of them before moving on to something else. Repetition after repetition always reaps the most rewards.

I was born and raised in Milwaukee, so I'm a big fan of the Green Bay Packers. Legendary football coach Vince Lombardi was well known for developing a play called the power sweep that became a staple of the Packers' championship-caliber offense in the 1960s. Lombardi's philosophy was to practice this single play over and over again until it was perfect. He often said that if everyone did his job, the running back should "run to daylight" and score every time. No, the Packers didn't score on every power sweep, but they got so good at running this one play that opposing defenses couldn't stop it even though they knew it was coming. The Packers committed to focusing on mastering fewer plays rather than being just okay at running a lot of plays, and this proved to be a winning strategy.

I want you to adopt this same winning strategy when it comes to the fitness program in this book: Focus on mastering fewer moves rather than being just okay at a lot of moves.

You'll end up burning more fat, building more muscle, and maximizing your physical performance at everything you do.

THE FOUR MOVEMENT CATEGORIES

It's one thing to focus on mastering fewer moves, but it's another thing to select the right movements to target. Rather than thinking about body parts, I want you to think about primal, natural, and athletic movement patterns that work multiple muscle groups at once. That creates efficiency and functional strength for everyday use. You can basically build a cutting-edge fitness program using only four distinct categories of movement: two for your lower body (hip dominant and knee dominant) and two for your upper body (pulling and pushing). Furthermore, within each movement category, there are two distinct exercises to master and switch between. This is the foundation of the Bodyweight 8 exercise system.

Here are the movement categories and corresponding exercises.

Lower-Body Movement Categories

Hip-Dominant Movements

These hip-centric movements revolve around the action of hinging (or bending) at your hips without moving your lower back and with minimal to no movement at your knees. Technically, these are lower-body pulling movements. They primarily work the muscles on the back side of your lower body (what exercise physiologists call the "posterior chain"), including your glutes, hamstrings, and spinal muscles. These muscles not only are the key to athletic performance but they are the most metabolically active muscles in your body. Translation:

They burn the most calories for every rep you do, and building them up to your potential will boost your metabolism so you burn more calories while at rest.

The two movements to master in this category are the Hip Thrust and Hip Hinge.

THE HIP THRUST (also know as Hip Extension or Glute Bridge) is a ground-based exercise popularized by top trainer Bret Contreras (better known as "the Glute Guy"). The action makes your glute muscles work hardest at terminal hip extension like no other exercise, making it arguably the best butt-building exercise on the planet.

THE HIP HINGE (also know as the Romanian Deadlift) is a standing exercise where you bend at your hips with a flat-back position; it will work your hamstrings and spinal muscles more than Hip Thrusts. It's also a more functional exercise because you're on your feet. The action requires more stability and flexibility to perform and will instantly make you a better squatter and athlete. You'll eventually perform this move on one leg at a time and achieve an elite level of balance and body awareness.

Being able to properly hinge at your hips is a prerequisite to properly performing the movements in the knee-dominant category. That's right: Using your hips more when you squat and lunge will not only make you stronger and more powerful but will also bulletproof your knees. That's why this movement category is so important, especially for people with a history of knee pain and lower-body injuries. In fact, many fitness experts recommend that most people perform 2 to 3 sets of hip-dominant movements for every set of knee-dominant movements they do. Whether you follow this prescription is up to you, but you at least want to make sure that you do an equal amount of both types of movements for structural balance and injury prevention.

Knee-Dominant Movements

These squat-centric movements revolve around bending at your knees and hips with a relatively upright body position. Technically, these are lower-body pushing movements. They primarily work the muscles on the front side of your lower body (what's known as the "anterior chain"), including your quads and hip flexors. When you do these movements correctly—that is, by initiating them through your hips instead of your knees—they also work your glutes and hamstrings in a serious way. Plus, when you perform these exercises through a full range of motion, you even work the calf and shin muscles of your lower legs.

The two movements to master in this category are the Deep Squat and Single-Leg Squat.

THE DEEP SQUAT is performed on both legs, and, obviously, Single-Leg Squats are performed on one leg at a time. If you want to be truly fit, you need to be able to do both very well. Deep Squats are tools to enhance your overall mobility and athleticism and will eventually be used to build pure power with explosive squat-jumping variations.

THE SINGLE-LEG SQUAT builds a sick amount of strength and stability. Both moves feed each other, and when combined, they will make you a squatter extraordinaire—and that's a very good thing. In addition, being able to properly squat sets the tone for how you do just about everything, like standing, walking, running, and even jumping. If you squat poorly (with your toes way out to the sides, your knees moving all over the place, and your back rounded), not only will your performance be piss-poor but you will set yourself up for some serious life-changing injuries.

Upper-Body Movement Categories
Pulling Movements

In these moves, you pull your body toward your hands. They primarily work the muscles on the back side of your upper body (posterior chain), including your lats, traps, rhomboids, and rear shoulders. They also work your biceps, forearms, and gripping muscles.

Many fitness experts recommend that most people would do well by performing 2 to 3 sets of upper-body pulling movements for every set of upper-body pushing movements they do. At the very least, you want to make sure that you do an equal amount of both types of movements for structural balance and injury prevention.

The two movements to master in this category are the Row and the Pullup.

THE ROW is a horizontal pulling pattern that works your upper-back/midback muscles.

THE PULLUP is a vertical pulling pattern that works your lats. Pullups are harder to do because you're lifting your entire body weight. However, Rows do a better job of working the entire back side of your body because your glutes, hamstrings, and spinal muscles need to engage and support your body throughout the movement.

Pushing Movements

In these moves, you push your body away from your hands. They primarily work the muscles on the front side of your upper body (anterior chain), including your chest and shoulders. They also work the back of your arms, or triceps. In addition, upper-body pushing movements require a lot of core stability and engage your abs from start to finish. Though there's nothing wrong with some isolated core work, rest assured that you'll give your abs all the work they need with Pushup variations. It's basically like holding a Plank position while moving your body up and down.

The two movements to master in this category are the Pushup and the Handstand Pushup.

THE PUSHUP is a horizontal pushing pattern that targets your chest.

THE HANDSTAND PUSHUP is a vertical pushing pattern that targets your shoulders. Handstand Pushups are harder to do because you're lifting your entire body weight. However, Pushups do a better job of working the entire front side of your body because your core, hip, and thigh muscles need to engage and support your body throughout the movement.

THE ECONOMICS OF EXERCISE

In college, I was a double major in economics and sociology. Pretty strange for a fitness guy, right? Well, I went to Amherst, a liberal arts college, and there were no classes offered for exercise science. So I decided to major in economics since I wanted to get into business and all of my buddies on the football team seemed to think it was a good idea. The sociology major was actually an accident, as I ended up taking just enough sociology classes to earn the major.

No disrespect intended to any economics enthusiasts, but I hated Econ. It just didn't resonate with me—all this theory with very little real-world application. I remember being so thrilled when I finally made it through microeconomics only to find that macroeconomics wasn't that much easier. That said, I did learn a valuable lesson that has helped me better formulate my system of exercise progressions.

You see, macroeconomics is the general study of the behavior of the economy as a whole, whereas microeconomics is the specific study of the behaviors of individuals and businesses. If you're already lost, don't worry! I'm still wrapping my head around all of that mess. What's important, however, is how this relates to fitness.

A macroexercise progression is a large vertical progression in which you're going from one level of difficulty to another. For example, moving from a Staggered Squat to a Lunge is a macroprogression. A microexercise progression is a small horizontal progression in which you're making a subtle modification to increase the challenge ever so slightly. For example, moving from a Reverse Lunge to a Forward Lunge is a microprogression. The big takeaway here is that macroprogressions involve a bigger jump in difficulty and microprogressions allow more modest jumps in difficulty, kind of like adding 5 pounds to a barbell.

Every exercise in the Bodyweight 8 program will have five distinct levels of difficulty that progressively take you from ground zero to superhero. On the next page are the macroprogressions for the Single-Leg Squat, as an example.

Within each level of difficulty will be three corresponding microregressions to make the move a bit easier and three corresponding microprogressions to make the move a bit harder. The importance of the microprogressions is that they allow you to completely customize your fitness experience. They show an advanced trainee how to make a ground zero exercise more challenging while making the superhero exercise accessible for even the novice trainee.

In addition, just because you progress past a certain level doesn't suddenly render that exercise useless or obsolete. Easier exercises can continue to be used during warmups or for active recovery between workouts. You can do them for higher reps to build endurance and burn more fat or even perform them explosively to build power and rapidly increase your heart rate.

Level 1	Level 2	Level 3	Level 4	Level 5
Ground Zero	Beginner	Intermediate	Advanced	Superhero
SINGLE-LEG WALL SIT	**STEPUP**	**STAGGERED SQUAT**	**LUNGE**	**SINGLE-LEG SQUAT**

THE GLOBAL CONCEPTS

Now that I've officially mortified and offended my economics professors, let's discuss some global concepts regarding proper exercise performance.

You'll see certain themes throughout this book. I call them global concepts. These four distinct concepts are essential for safe and efficient exercise performance and, when internalized, will be the key to longevity in the fitness arena. They will instantly enhance your performance and reduce your risk of injury.

❶ **Tripod foot position**

❷ **Hollow-body position**

❸ **Diaphragmatic breathing (belly breathing)**

❹ **Stable hip and shoulder position**

Tripod Foot Position

You probably never considered this unless you're a runner, but maintaining a natural arch in your foot is critical to your overall health and performance. Many people struggle to load either point of their forefoot: the knuckle of the big toe (first metatarsal head) or the knuckle of the little toe (fifth metatarsal head). If you put too much weight on the knuckle of your big toe, then your arch will collapse and your foot will roll inward, known as overpronation. If you put too much weight on the knuckle of your little toe, then your foot will roll to the outside, known as oversupination. Both actions result in an unstable foot that will wreak havoc up your kinetic chain. That's where the tripod foot position comes into play for the purpose of performing the exercises in this book.

In tripod foot position, your weight is evenly distributed on three parts of your foot: the knuckle of your big toe, the knuckle of your little toe, and your heel.

To properly set up in the tripod foot position, first lift your toes off the ground. This will make it easier for you to find the three key points of contact. Then, slowly lower your toes to the ground without losing the ground contact and even weight distribution of the tripod foot. Balance here for a moment, and then progress to balancing on one leg. Your ultimate goal is to be able to hold this single-leg balance position for at least a minute without allowing the other foot to touch the ground. You can make it more challenging by moving your head and looking around, by closing your eyes, or by adding movement of your arms and nonworking leg.

The tripod foot position is the foundation of all standing exercises, particularly those for the lower body. It will make you a great squatter and ultimately a great athlete, and, most important, it will save your knees! Work these single-leg balance drills into your warmups, and take the time to carefully set up your tripod foot position before every work set for best results.

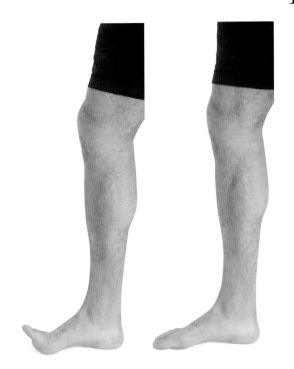

BEST WORKOUT SHOES

Most shoes elevate your heels and compress your toes, which makes it very difficult to execute tripod foot position. That's why I advocate training barefoot or while wearing a minimalist workout shoe with a wider toe box and minimal heel elevation that keeps your feet closer to the floor. My three favorites are:

XERO SHOES. Like an extreme fitness sandal, these are as close to barefoot as you can get. They provide nice traction for ground contact, which is important for people like me with very sweaty feet. A strap encases the top of the foot and the heel for structure and support. This shoe is best for static and linear movements like walking and running; it is not ideal for explosive, multidirectional movements because of the lack of lateral stability.

NEW BALANCE MINIMUS SERIES. My favorite minimalist cross-training shoe is the Minimus 20v3. It has just enough cushioning to absorb impact on harder surfaces, and the toe box is super wide and comfortable. I even play full-court basketball several times per week in these shoes without worry of turning an ankle because they keep my foot low.

VIBRAM FIVEFINGERS. This is what most people consider to be the original barefoot shoe. It is super close to the ground and sports individual "fingers" for each of your five toes. I love using these shoes for my bodyweight workouts, but they don't have a lot of cushioning for more explosive movements on harder surfaces.

Hollow-Body Position

One of the foundational positions in gymnastics is called the hollow body. It's one of the first a young gymnast learns because it's integral to many other movements. The Hollow-Body Hold is an exercise in abdominal bracing and total-body tension that will allow you to properly transfer force from your upper body to your lower body without any energy leaks in the kinetic chain.

The hollow-body position is easiest to learn standing on your feet. Here's how to do it.

- Establish tripod foot position.

- Place your feet together.

- Squeeze your legs together.

- Tense your thighs.

- Clench your glutes.

- Brace your abs.

- Push your ribs and shoulders down.

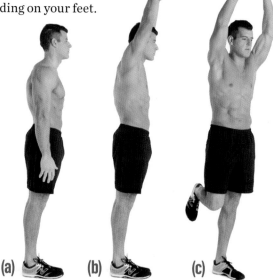

Start with your arms at your sides (a) and then increase the challenge by raising your arms overhead without letting your positioning change (b). From, there maintain this position while standing on one leg (c).

From there, progress to a Lying Hollow-Body Hold with your back on the floor. It's like performing a Plank while lying on your back, and it will improve your performance on Pushups, Pullups, and Single-Leg Squats.

Here's how to do it.

- Lie on your back and place your feet together and point your toes away from your body.

- Press your tongue into the roof of your mouth to engage your neck stabilizers.

- Squeeze your legs together, and tense your thighs.

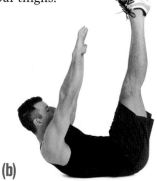

LYING HOLLOW-BODY HOLD

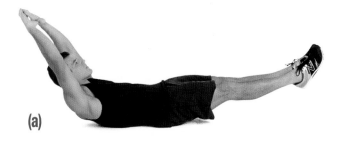

- Raise your arms overhead.

- Clench your glutes.

- Brace your abs.

- Push your ribs and shoulders down.

- Now raise your head, arms, shoulders, and legs off the floor and hold for time (a). This great move stabilizes the low back. If it's too challenging, regress it by raising your arms and legs higher until they are close together as shown (b).

The key to doing this exercise correctly is maintaining a posterior pelvic tilt, in which your abs are crunched and braced and your lower back is firmly compressed into the floor. Do not hyperextend the lumbar spine. There should be no space between your lower back and the floor. For this reason, the hollow is unmatched for bulletproofing your back and sculpting your abs. It also sets the tone for perfect posture, teaching you an abdominal bracing strategy that can be employed while seated, standing, or lying down.

Master the basic hollow hold, holding for 30 to 60 seconds at a time. Your whole body will work harder to stay tight and together and prevent unwanted motion at your spine.

Another great variation is the Hollow-Body Bridge Hold. This move works your entire back side and is the perfect companion to the hollow hold. Maintain that posterior pelvic tilt with your abs crunched as if bracing for a punch to your gut. The movement is slight, as you will lift your hips only a couple inches off of the floor while maintaining ground contact with your feet, shoulders, and head (a). Your feet can be spaced wider apart with this variation, if you'd like. You should instantly feel it in your hips and hamstrings. Make it harder by picking up one leg at a time (b) or by extending your arms overhead (c).

One of my favorite 5-minute core workouts is switching between a Lying Hollow-Body Hold and a Lying Hollow-Body Bridge Hold every 30 seconds with no rest in between. Do it for 10 straight minutes if you want your core to feel like Mike Tyson went 15 rounds on your midsection.

You can add these hollow-body moves to your warmup or as a core exercise within a total-body workout. Because they emphasize posture, you can also do them daily without fear of overtraining. The key takeaway here is that you know that whenever I say "assume the hollow-body position," it means:

- Squeeze your legs together.

- Tense your thighs.

- Clench your glutes.

- Brace your abs.

- Push your ribs and shoulders down.

- Keep your head in a neutral position, with your ears aligned directly over your shoulders, hips, and ankles.

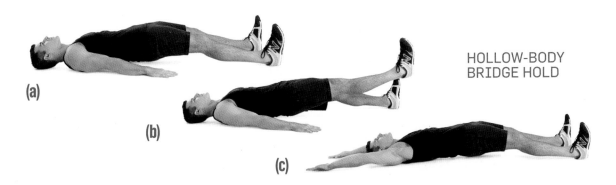

(a)

(b)

(c)

HOLLOW-BODY BRIDGE HOLD

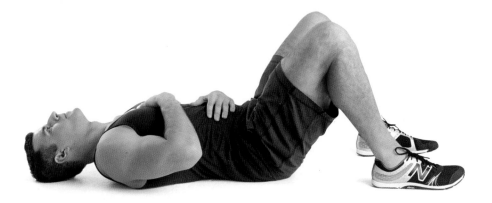

Diaphragmatic Breathing

Too many people breathe from their chests instead of their bellies. Test yourself. Stand and place one hand on your chest and the other on your belly. Breathe normally. Does your rib cage expand and rise? Are your shoulder blades rising toward your ears? That's chest breathing, and it will put your back and shoulders at risk of injury.

Belly breathing, or diaphragmatic breathing, is when your belly rises before your chest does. Diaphragmatic breathing can improve joint range of motion, boost exercise performance, decrease the risk of injury, and delay fatigue during activities with a high cardio-respiratory demand.

Here's how to practice.

- Lie on your back and place one hand on your belly and the other on your chest.

- Now do a series of deep inhales and exhales through your belly; 5 to 10 reps are ideal.

- You should feel your belly rise before your chest does.

Once you've got the belly breathing down while lying on the floor in a relaxed state, try to employ belly breathing in the hollow-body position. Maintaining total-body tension and a braced core increases the difficulty of breathing through your belly, so it's a natural progression. Keep in mind that with enough cardiovascular demand and metabolic stress, at some point your body will be forced to revert to some chest breathing. The goal here is simply to breathe through your belly as much as possible and prolong the amount of time you can do so before your other respiratory muscles kick in for assistance.

If you find belly breathing to be a bit confusing or tough to do, especially during exercise, don't sweat it too much. As long as you can brace your core properly, as seen with the hollow-body position mentioned earlier, your breathing will regulate itself.

Stable Hip and Shoulder Position

"It's all in the hips, it's all in the hips, it's all in the hips. . . ."

This is one of the more unforgettable lines from the cult classic movie *Happy Gilmore* where former pro golfer Chubbs Peterson (played by Carl Weathers, the same guy who played Apollo in *Rocky*) teaches Happy Gilmore (Adam Sandler), a former hockey player, how to swing a golf club. Well, I couldn't agree more. Except, I would update that statement to say:

"It's all in the hips *and* shoulders."

The hips and shoulders are the host sites to the most muscular and metabolically active areas in your body. As a result, they have the biggest impact on your overall exercise performance and metabolic rate. If you're looking to burn the most fat and calories during and after your workouts, then you need to get both your hips and shoulders on board every time you train.

Second, most lower-body movements are driven through your hips, and most upper-body movements are driven through your shoulders. With all of this driving going on, the hips and shoulders get a lot of miles put on them, so it's critical that you get these babies in a safe and stable position.

The hips and shoulders are ball-and-socket joints that allow you to get full rotational movement at your legs and arms, respectively. With this movement comes great responsibility, because motion without stability is a recipe for joint demolition. All you need to know is that to make these critical joints stable, you

must create external rotation torque to spiral these suckers into their sockets.

These coaching cues create an external rotation force that spirals your hips into their sockets for ultimate stability and strength.

- Maintain the tripod foot position.
- Keep your toes pointing as straight ahead as possible.
- Stomp and screw your feet into the floor.
- Push the floor apart with your feet.
- Push your knees out.
- Keep your shins as vertical as possible.

These coaching cues create an external rotation force that spirals your shoulders into their sockets.

- Push the floor apart with your hands when pushing.
- Pull the bar apart with your hands when pulling.
- Hug your elbows tight to your rib cage.
- Keep your armpits forward when your arms are overhead.
- Keep your elbow pits forward when your arms are in front of your body.
- Keep your forearms as vertical as possible.

If you embrace these performance pointers, you will absolutely dominate the exercises and workouts in this book, and your joints will be supple to boot. Now it's time to get the exercises!

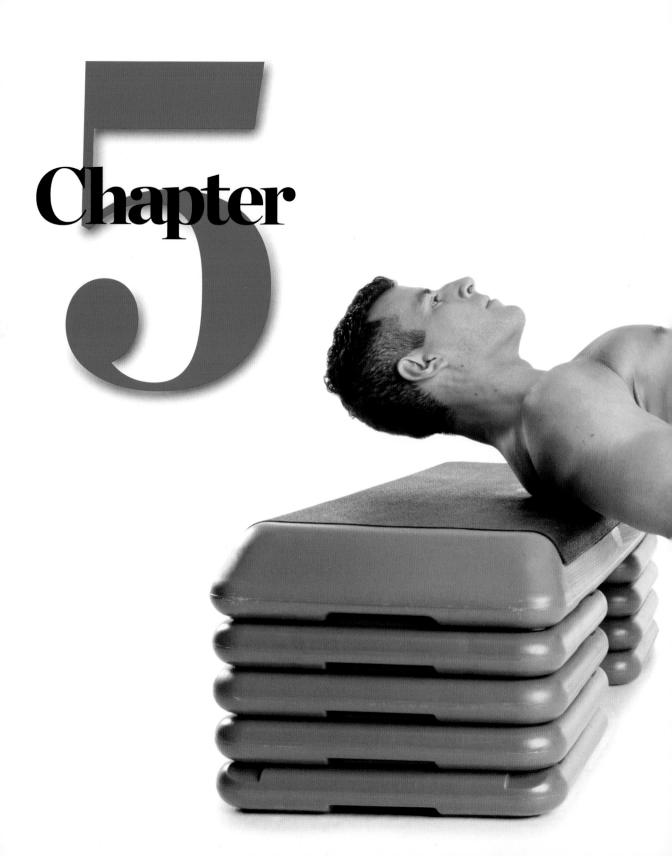

Chapter 5

BODYWEIGHT 8: HIP THRUST

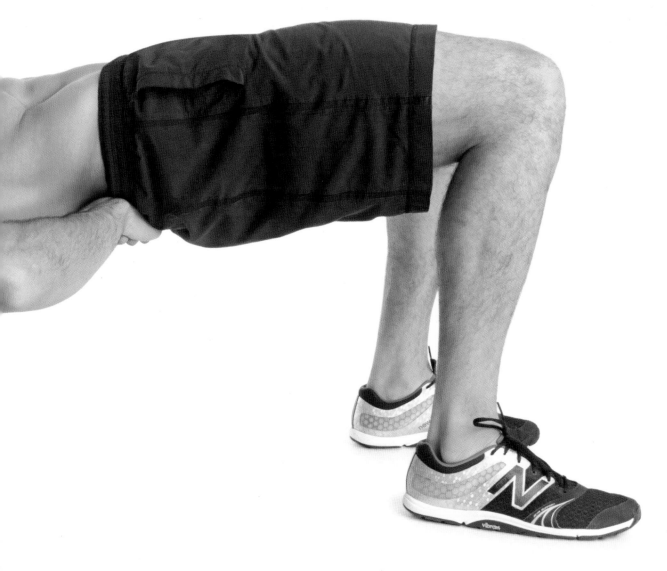

#1 HIP THRUST

There is no more important muscle group in your body than your glutes, or your butt muscles. They are your biggest and most powerful muscles, and they contract to move your hips in every which way, driving every activity. Because they are so large, they have the biggest potential impact on your metabolic rate. Develop them well, and you'll become more athletic and burn more calories 24-7. Unfortunately, most people's glutes are doing a disappearing act that would make Houdini envious. Here's why....

We spend most of our day sitting, which causes the muscles in front of our hips to shorten and tighten. Also, bloodflow becomes restricted, limiting the delivery of oxygen and nutrients to the area and clouding the communication between your brain and butt. The result? Your glute muscles stop firing. Fitness experts call this "gluteal amnesia." Over time, it makes your glutes wither away like melting glaciers. You'll be left with a butt that curves in instead of out, and your hips will be so weak that your knees and back have to pick up the slack for your gluteal delinquency. That makes your knees and back ache. You have a new appreciation for your ass now, don't you?

Well, there is no better exercise to turn your glutes on and open up your hips than the Hip Thrust. It's super safe to practice and incredibly easy to learn. You can do a version of it anytime, anywhere, even in a chair at your desk, on the couch while you're watching TV, or in an airplane seat when traveling. For optimal health and performance, hold the top position of one of these Hip Thrust variations for at least 20 seconds for every 20 minutes that you're in a seated position during the day. Sure, you're going to look like you're humping the air, but there's nothing wrong with becoming a highly proficient pelvic thruster. I often say that the glutes are like hot dogs—they plump when you cook 'em—and we're gonna be cooking those butt cheeks in a serious way.

The HIP THRUST Progression

Level 1	Level 2	Level 3	Level 4	Level 5
Ground Zero	Beginner	Intermediate	Advanced	Superhero
HIP THRUST	SHOULDERS-ELEVATED HIP THRUST	FEET-ELEVATED HIP THRUST	SHOULDERS-AND FEET-ELEVATED HIP THRUST	SINGLE-LEG HIP THRUST

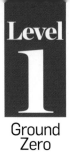

HIP THRUST

This entry-level Hip Thrust is a bridging exercise, basically a Plank for the back side of your body. The key is to maintain what's called a posterior pelvic tilt throughout the exercise by bracing your core and tilting your pelvis backward. The best way to ensure you nail this position is to start the movement with your lower back fully compressed into the floor with no daylight sneaking in under your spine. This keeps your lower back fixed and forces all of the movement to come through your hips. If you feel pain or discomfort in your lower back as your hips rise upward, it's probably because you're hyperextending your lower back. Fix that!

Hand placement: Place your hands on the floor with your palms up or down. The palms-facing-up version has the added benefit of externally rotating your shoulders and activating the muscles of your rear shoulders and upper back to correct the poor rounded-shoulders posture. You can also place the back of your hands on your lower back while performing the movement to rotate your shoulders internally, stretch your chest, and help you notice when you are overextending your lower back.

Foot placement: You can perform the Hip Thrust on your toes, on your heels, or with feet flat on the floor to work different muscles.

How to Do It

Starting Position

• Lie on your back with your knees bent at 90-degree angles.

• Place your feet flat on the floor hip-width apart.

• Keep your weight placed in the center of your feet (in front of your anklebone).

Perfect Execution

• First, crunch your abs and tilt your pelvis back so that your lower back is flat against the floor. You must maintain this posterior pelvic tilt throughout the duration of the exercise.

• Then push through your feet and raise your hips as high as you can without arching your lower back.

• Briefly hold this top position and then slowly reverse the movement and repeat.

Your Goal

You should be able to perform multiple sets of 10 reps, maintaining a straight torso line from your knees through your shoulders while in the top position.

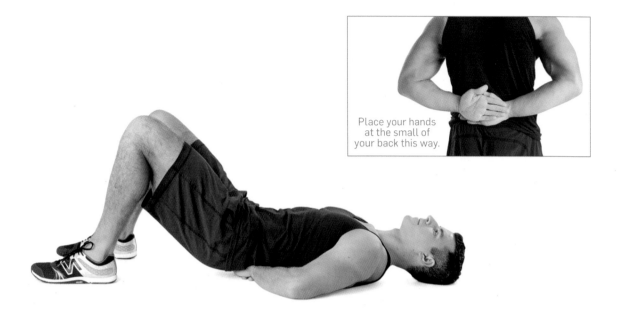

Place your hands at the small of your back this way.

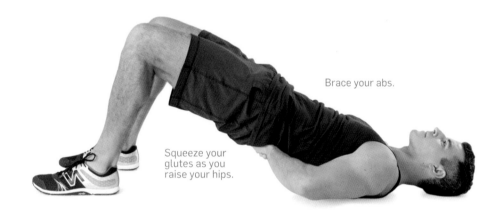

Brace your abs.

Squeeze your glutes as you raise your hips.

Regressions

MAKE IT EASIER: Hold the top position isometrically for time.

EVEN EASIER: Move your feet wider apart to increase your base of support.

EASIEST: Perform Self-Assisted Hip Thrusts by placing your hands on your butt and pushing your hips up with your hands.

Progressions

MAKE IT HARDER: Reduce your base of support by holding your hands at your sides so that only the backs of your upper arms are making contact with the ground.

EVEN HARDER: Further reduce your base of support by placing your fingertips on your forehead or by crossing your arms and grasping your shoulders.

HARDEST: Increase the range of motion by bringing your feet closer together until they touch.

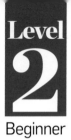

SHOULDERS-ELEVATED HIP THRUST

Elevating your shoulders on a stable box or bench allows you to increase the range of motion at your hips, provides a greater challenge for your quads (making it a great move to protect your knees and complement your Squats), and results in maximum glute activation to build your butt better. That's why top trainer and Hip Thrust enthusiast Bret Contreras calls this exercise "the Bench Press for your butt." The ideal height for shoulder elevation is one where your trunk forms a 45-degree angle with the floor, with your hips resting on or hovering just above the ground in the down position, and where knees and shoulders are directly aligned in the top position.

How to Do It

Starting Position

- Place your upper back/midback on a stable box or bench with your arms at your sides and hands on the small of your back.
- Place your feet flat on the floor and hip-width apart.
- Keep your weight placed in the center of your feet (in front of your anklebone).

Perfect Execution

- First, crunch your abs and tilt your pelvis back so that your lower back is flat. You must maintain this posterior pelvic tilt throughout the exercise.
- Then push through your feet and raise your hips as high as you can without extending your lower back.
- Briefly hold this top position and then slowly reverse the movement and repeat.

Your Goal

You should be able to perform multiple sets of 10 reps, maintaining a straight line from your knees through your shoulders while in the top position.

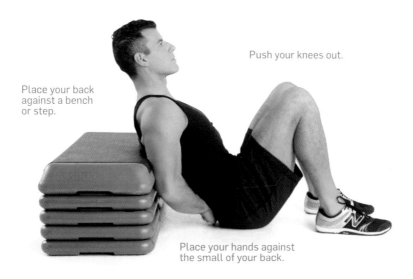

Push your knees out.

Place your back against a bench or step.

Place your hands against the small of your back.

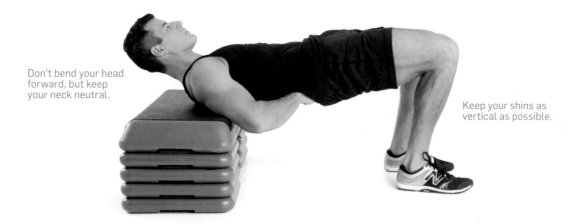

Don't bend your head forward, but keep your neck neutral.

Keep your shins as vertical as possible.

Regressions

MAKE IT EASIER: Hold the top position isometrically for time.

EVEN EASIER: Increase your base of support and decrease the range of motion by widening your foot placement.

EASIEST: Perform Self-Assisted Hip Thrusts by placing your hands on your butt and pushing your hips up as much as needed to achieve full hip extension without moving your lower back.

Progressions

MAKE IT HARDER: Reduce your base of support by holding your hands at your sides so that only the backs of your upper arms are making contact.

EVEN HARDER: Further reduce your base of support by placing your fingertips on your forehead or by crossing your arms so that each hand is placed on the opposite shoulder.

HARDEST: Increase the range of motion by bringing your feet closer together until they are touching.

FEET-ELEVATED HIP THRUST

Elevating your feet on a stable box or bench tests your hamstrings because your hips drop below the level of your feet. This makes your hamstrings work double duty by having to both bend your knees and extend your hips. Exercising both functions of your hamstrings will provide the most complete development for your rear thighs and make you a better runner. Strong hamstrings are critical to knee health, and when they can work in perfect concert with your glutes, they'll deliver some serious horsepower. Another cool benefit is that well-built hamstrings make your legs look really attractive when viewed from the side. The optimal height to elevate your feet is about the same as with the Shoulders-Elevated Hip Thrust.

How to Do It

Starting Position

• Lie on your back and place your feet on a stable box, bench, or chair.

• Your hips should be a couple inches in front of the elevated surface.

• Keep your weight in the center of your feet (in front of your anklebone).

Perfect Execution

• First, crunch your abs and tilt your pelvis back so that your lower back is flat. Maintain this posterior pelvic tilt throughout the exercise.

• Then push through your feet and raise your hips as high as you can without extending your lower back.

• Briefly hold this top position and then slowly reverse the movement and repeat.

Your Goal

You should be able to perform multiple sets of 10 reps, maintaining a straight line from your knees through your shoulders while in the top position.

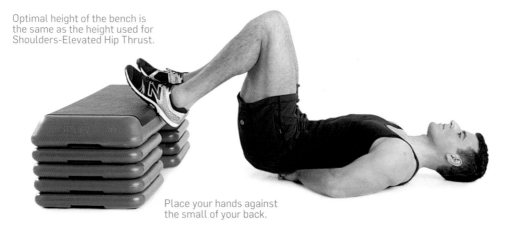

Optimal height of the bench is the same as the height used for Shoulders-Elevated Hip Thrust.

Place your hands against the small of your back.

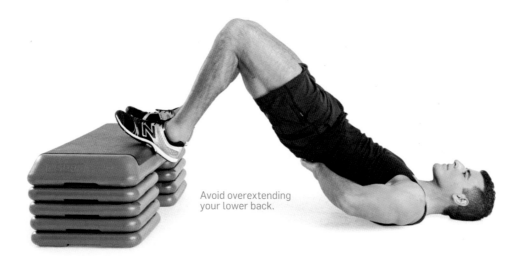

Avoid overextending your lower back.

Regressions

MAKE IT EASIER: Hold the top position isometrically for time.

EVEN EASIER: Increase your base of support and decrease the range of motion by widening your foot placement.

EASIEST: Perform Self-Assisted Hip Thrusts by placing your hands on your butt and pushing your hips up with your hands.

Progressions

MAKE IT HARDER: Hold your hands against your sides so that only the backs of your upper arms are in contact with the ground.

EVEN HARDER: Further reduce your base of support by placing your fingertips on your forehead or by crossing your arms so that each hand is on the opposite shoulder.

HARDEST: Increase the range of motion by bringing your feet closer together until they touch.

SHOULDERS- AND FEET- ELEVATED HIP THRUST

This is the most challenging Hip Thrust variation on two legs because it takes your hips through the greatest range of motion. In most cases, your shoulders and feet should be elevated at the same level, if possible. Having your shoulders elevated higher than your feet will shift more work to your quads. Having your feet elevated higher than your shoulders will shift more work to your hamstrings. Again, all are good options, so feel free to mix and match.

How to Do It

Starting Position

• Place your upper back/midback and hands on a stable box, bench, or chair, with your arms extended out to your sides on top of the step for support (not shown).

• Place your feet on another bench of similar height that is about 3 feet away.

• Raise your butt an inch above the floor.

Perfect Execution

• Keeping your back flat, push through your feet, and raise your hips as high as you can without extending your lower back.

• Briefly hold this top position and then slowly reverse the movement and repeat.

Your Goal

You should be able to perform multiple sets of 10 reps, maintaining a straight line from your knees through your shoulders while in the top position.

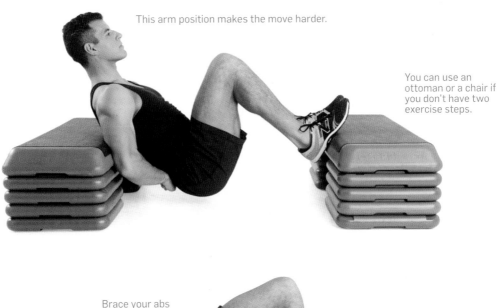

This arm position makes the move harder.

You can use an ottoman or a chair if you don't have two exercise steps.

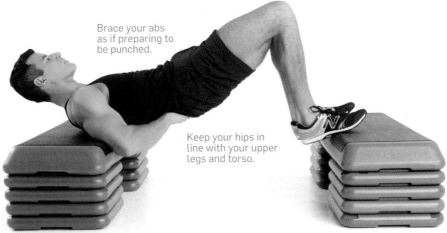

Brace your abs as if preparing to be punched.

Keep your hips in line with your upper legs and torso.

Regressions

MAKE IT EASIER: Simply hold the top position isometrically for time.

EVEN EASIER: Increase your base of support by widening your foot placement.

EASIEST: Perform Self-Assisted Hip Thrusts by placing your hands on your butt and pushing your hips up as much as needed to achieve full hip extension without moving your lower back.

Progressions

MAKE IT HARDER: Reduce your base of support by lifting your arms off the elevated surface so that only the backs of your arms are making contact.

EVEN HARDER: Further reduce your base of support by placing your fingertips on your forehead or by crossing your arms so that each hand is placed on the opposite shoulder.

HARDEST: Increase the range of motion by bringing your feet closer together until they touch.

SINGLE-LEG HIP THRUST

This is the granddaddy of them all. Lifting your hips one leg at a time requires a great deal of hip stability and strength. It will also help you iron out any strength and flexibility imbalances between sides of your glutes and hips. The Single-Leg Hip Thrust is the ultimate companion exercise to the Single-Leg Squat (see Chapter 11) because it builds the prerequisite backside strength, core stability, and hip mobility needed to pull that movement off. If you have a history of knee and back pain, this move should be a staple of your weekly training routine. Plus, this is the one move that most people with lower-body injuries are still able to perform pain-free, making it great for rehabilitation.

How to Do It

Starting Position

• Lie on your back with the foot of your working leg placed flat on the floor and underneath your knee so that it's bent at a 90-degree angle.

• Bend the knee of your nonworking leg toward your chest without moving your lower back.

• Keep your weight in the center of the foot of your working leg (in front of your anklebone).

Perfect Execution

• First, crunch your abs and tilt your pelvis back so that your lower back is flattened against your hands or the floor. Maintain this posterior pelvic tilt throughout the exercise.

• Push through the foot on the floor and raise your hips as high as you can without extending your lower back.

• Briefly hold this top position and then slowly reverse the movement and repeat.

Your Goal

You should be able to perform multiple sets of 10 reps per side, maintaining a straight line from your knees through your shoulders while in the top position.

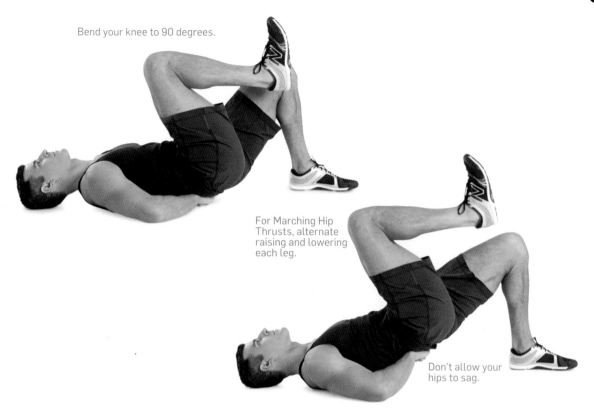

Bend your knee to 90 degrees.

For Marching Hip Thrusts, alternate raising and lowering each leg.

Don't allow your hips to sag.

Regressions

MAKE IT EASIER: Place the foot of your nonworking leg on top of your working leg just above the knee. The knee of the nonworking leg should be bent at a 90-degree angle.

EVEN EASIER: Perform Marching Hip Thrusts by slowly alternating legs every couple seconds while holding the top Hip Thrust position for the full duration of the exercise.

EASIEST: Perform Gyrating Hip Thrusts. Place both feet on the floor with knees bent and slowly shift your pelvis side to side to make one glute work harder than the other.

Progressions

MAKE IT HARDER: Perform Single-Leg Hip Thrusts with your shoulders elevated on a bench.

EVEN HARDER: Perform Single-Leg Hip Thrusts with your feet elevated on a bench.

HARDEST: Perform Single-Leg Hip Thrusts with your shoulders *and* feet elevated.

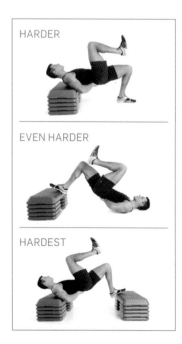

HARDER

EVEN HARDER

HARDEST

Variations

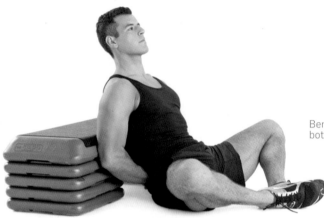

Bend your knees and place the bottoms of your feet together.

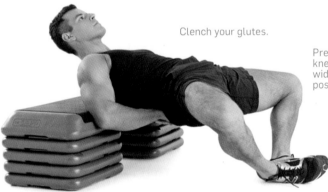

Clench your glutes.

Press your knees out as wide as possible.

1. Externally Rotated Hip Thrust—Knees Out

Your butt is made up of three muscles, the gluteus maximus, medius, and minimus. Maximus lifts your hips; medius and minimus provide lateral and rotational hip movement. This variation works all three muscles. It loosens tight groin muscles and improves your ability to get your knees out when squatting. Place the bottoms of your feet together and push your knees out as far as you can, like an open clamshell, while squeezing your outer hips.

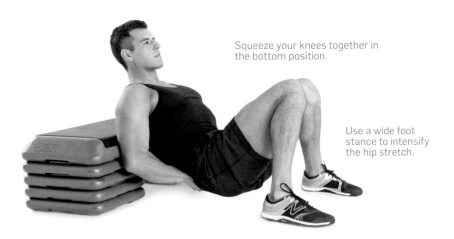

Squeeze your knees together in the bottom position.

Use a wide foot stance to intensify the hip stretch.

Press your knees out to shoulder width in the top position.

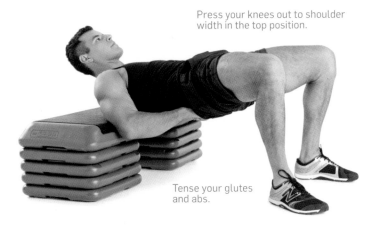

Tense your glutes and abs.

2. Internally Rotated Hip Thrust—Knees In

Perform Hip Thrusts with your knees touching when in the bottom position and out as normal during the thrust. The wider your foot placement, the harder it will be to get your knees together and the more intense the stretch. This variation will improve your internal hip rotation and make it easier for you to keep your toes pointing straight ahead when standing, walking, and squatting.

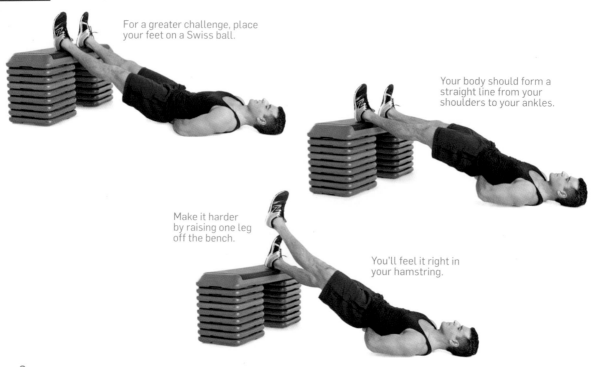

For a greater challenge, place your feet on a Swiss ball.

Your body should form a straight line from your shoulders to your ankles.

Make it harder by raising one leg off the bench.

You'll feel it right in your hamstring.

3. Straight-Leg Hip Thrust with Feet Elevated

You've learned to do Hip Thrusts with knees bent. In this movement, also known as the Hollow-Body Bridge Hold (see page 41), you thrust with legs straight, which forces your hamstrings to work harder to lift your hips and calls on your hips and abs to stabilize your spine.

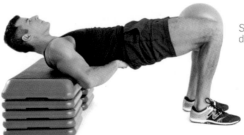

Squeeze your knees; don't let the ball drop.

4. Squeezing Hip Thrust

Squeeze a ball, foam roller, rolled-up towel, or the head of your arch nemesis between your legs while doing Hip Thrusts. This will activate all of the muscles of your pelvic floor, providing even greater stability to your lower back.

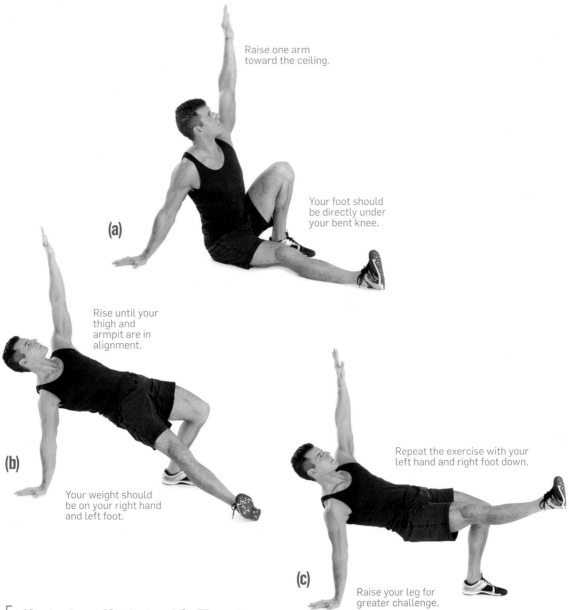

Raise one arm toward the ceiling.

Your foot should be directly under your bent knee.

(a)

Rise until your thigh and armpit are in alignment.

(b)

Your weight should be on your right hand and left foot.

Repeat the exercise with your left hand and right foot down.

(c)

Raise your leg for greater challenge.

5. Single-Arm, Single-Leg Hip Thrust

Place your right hand on the floor with your right foot fully extended in front of your body, the leg resting on the floor. Place your left foot on the floor so it's positioned directly underneath your left knee and raise your left arm (a). Now drive through your left foot and extend your hips as high as you can without moving your lower back (b). Pause briefly, reverse the movement, and repeat. Make it harder by keeping the nonworking leg elevated throughout the duration of the exercise (c).

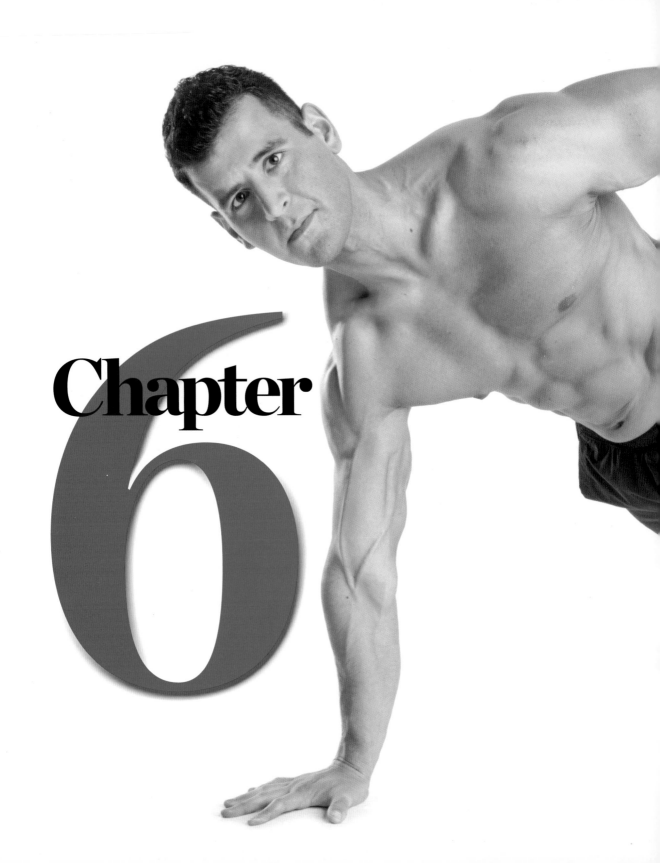

Chapter 6

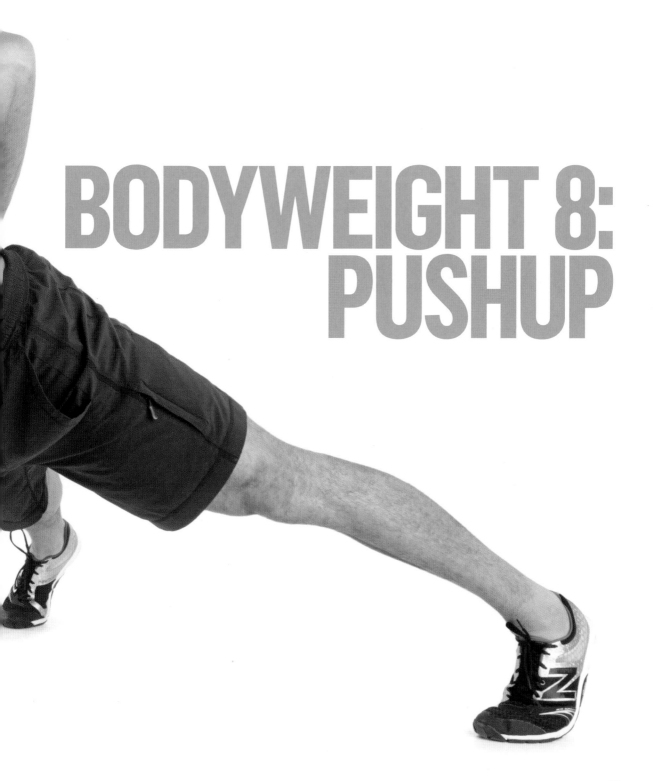

BODYWEIGHT 8: PUSHUP

#2
PUSHUP

When most people think about exercise, the first move that comes to mind is the Pushup, the iconic Rocky Balboa move (he did it on one arm, not two) that continues to inspire generations of people to get off of the couch and get down to fighting weight. It's a classic calisthenics exercise that has been used for centuries to build strong upper bodies; supple wrist, elbow, and shoulder joints; and primal punching and pushing power. There are probably more ways to do Pushups than just about any other exercise, giving you a lifetime of variety and results.

The Pushup is to the upper body what the Squat is to the lower body. While the Squat teaches you how to create a stable hip position, the Pushup teaches you how to create a stable shoulder position. When done correctly, both exercises engage nearly every muscle in your body, giving you a nearly complete fitness program. No two other exercises can combine for such an effective and versatile anytime, anywhere total-body workout.

The Pushup is a superior exercise to the Bench Press (or Chest Press) for several reasons. First of all, it works your chest, front shoulders, and triceps just as hard as a Bench Press will as long as you train the Pushup progressively. Second, the Pushup forces you to support your entire body in a Plank position, working all of the muscles on the front side of your body (plus many on the back side), while the Bench Press has you lying on your back. As a result, every rep of the Pushup works more muscles and burns more calories than every rep of the Bench Press. What's more, each Pushup progression demands more from your abs to maintain stability. When you reach the Single-Arm Pushup level, you'll be performing the best abdominal exercise you can do because it requires your core to stabilize your spine in all three planes of motion.

The PUSHUP Progression

Level 1	Level 2	Level 3	Level 4	Level 5
Ground Zero	Beginner	Intermediate	Advanced	Superhero
PLANK	PUSHUP	SELF-ASSISTED SINGLE-ARM PUSHUP	SINGLE-ARM PUSHUP	PLYOMETRIC PUSHUP

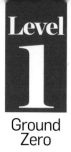

PLANK

The foundation of a perfect Pushup is being able to hold a hollow-body position at the top of the movement with your arms fully extended. This is also called planking. Planks will ensure that you build the core and shoulder stability needed to execute full-range-of-motion Pushups. A strong, braced core allows you to properly align your ribs and pelvis so that your hips and shoulders travel together as one unit with no wasted movement or energy leaks in the kinetic chain. In fact, you should be able to plank a level or two higher than your current Pushup level. For example, you should be able to plank on one leg or one arm or with your feet elevated before doing a regular floor Pushup. This will ensure that your core is always up for the task so you can focus on pushing instead of stabilizing.

Keep your feet together as much as possible throughout these progressions. Though it gives you a smaller support base, keeping your feet together makes it much easier for you to engage your hip and core muscles to lock in a neutral spine position with a slight arch in your lower back.

How to Do It

Starting Position

- Place your hands directly underneath your shoulders with your arms extended.
- Keep your weight over the center of your hands (just in front of your wrists).
- Screw your hands into the floor and grip the ground with your fingertips.
- Spread your fingertips as wide as you can.
- Set your head in a neutral position with your ears aligned with your shoulders, hips, and ankles, and look between your hands.
- Assume a hollow-body position: Squeeze your legs together, tense your thighs, glutes, and abs, and pull your ribs and shoulders down.

Perfect Execution

- Hold this Plank position for time while actively maintaining hollow-body mechanics for the duration of the exercise.
- Focus on deep belly breathing.

Your Goal

You should be able to perform multiple sets of 60-second holds before moving to the next level.

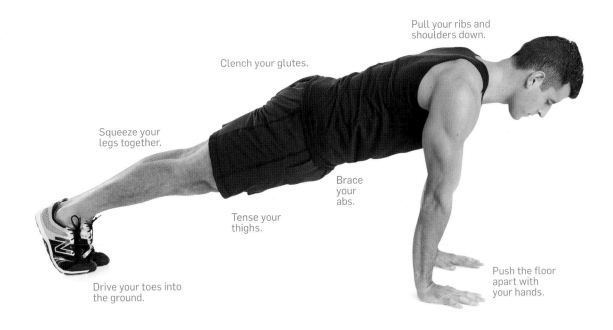

Pull your ribs and shoulders down.

Clench your glutes.

Squeeze your legs together.

Brace your abs.

Tense your thighs.

Drive your toes into the ground.

Push the floor apart with your hands.

Regressions

MAKE IT EASIER: Increase your base of support by widening your hands and feet as much as needed.

EVEN EASIER: Break up a longer hold into shorter 5- to 10-second holds with brief 2- to 5-second rest periods. Gradually lengthen each hold and take less rest.

EASIEST: Decrease your body angle by performing a Hands-Elevated Plank. Place your hands (or forearms) on a sturdy box, bench, or chair. This makes it much easier because you're holding less of your body weight.

Progressions

MAKE IT HARDER: Lift one leg off the floor and focus on squeezing the glute of your supporting leg. Or progressively bring your hands together until your thumbs touch.

EVEN HARDER: Lift a hand off the floor and extend that arm in front of you. Widen your feet to help balance.

HARDEST: Raise a leg and the opposing arm off the floor to hold your body weight with only two points of floor contact.

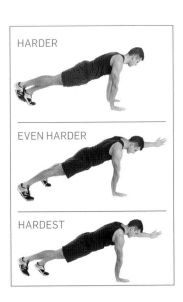

HARDER

EVEN HARDER

HARDEST

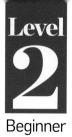

PUSHUP

You've been doing Pushups since elementary school PE, but are you doing them properly? For pecs that pop, you will want to perform a mix of different body angles, hand positions, and dynamic full-range-of-motion repetitions. If you want big arms, you need to pay attention to your triceps—after all, they comprise approximately two-thirds of your upper arms. Work your triceps by bringing your hands closer together until your thumbs are touching. The close grip increases elbow range of motion, which will help prep your triceps and elbows for the demands of the Single-Arm Pushup.

At the top of each Pushup, be sure to push away your shoulder blades while keeping your chest out. Doing so will put extra stress on the muscle positioned just alongside your rib cage, the serratus anterior, also known as the puncher's muscle because it's usually well developed in boxers.

How to Do It

Starting Position

- Place your hands directly underneath your shoulders with arms fully extended.
- Keep your weight over the center of your hands.
- Screw your hands into the floor and grip the ground with your fingertips.
- Spread your fingertips as wide as you can.
- Assume a hollow-body position: Squeeze your legs together, tense your thighs, glutes, and abs, and pull your ribs and shoulders down.

Perfect Execution

- Tuck your elbows to your sides and slowly pull yourself into the bottom position until your chest hovers just above the floor.
- Hold this bottom position briefly and squeeze your shoulder blades together.
- Then reverse the movement, being sure to fully extend your arms, and push your shoulder blades away from each other at the top of the movement.

Your Goal

You should be able to perform multiple sets of 10 reps before moving to the next level.

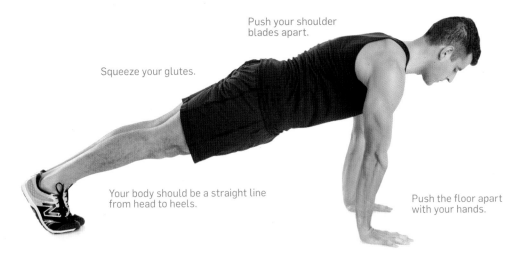

Push your shoulder blades apart.

Squeeze your glutes.

Your body should be a straight line from head to heels.

Push the floor apart with your hands.

Tuck your elbows.

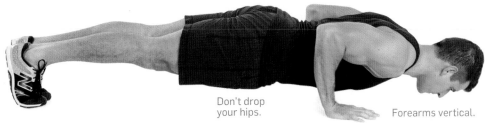

Don't drop your hips.

Forearms vertical.

Regressions

MAKE IT EASIER: Perform Eccentric Pushups by only doing the lowering portion of the exercise (take at least 3 to 5 seconds to lower). Cheat back up by using your knees.

EVEN EASIER: Perform Isometric Pushups by holding the bottom (or top) position for time.

EASIEST: Place your hands on a sturdy box, bench, or chair. This makes it much easier because you're pushing less of your body weight. Elevate your hands as much as needed in order to be able to perform full-range-of-motion Pushups. Gradually work your way down to the floor by decreasing the elevation height.

Progressions

MAKE IT HARDER: Lift one leg off the floor and focus on squeezing the glute of your supporting leg.

EVEN HARDER: Perform Close-Grip Pushups by progressively narrowing your hand placement until the thumbs of your hands are touching. You could also increase the range of motion by placing your hands on elevated boxes, books, balls, or weight plates of even height. This will allow your chest to sink lower than the floor would allow.

HARDEST: Place your feet on a sturdy box, bench, or chair. This makes it much harder because you're pushing more of your body weight.

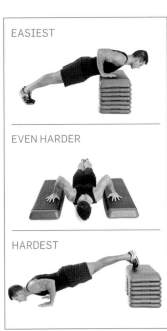

EASIEST

EVEN HARDER

HARDEST

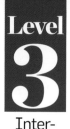
SELF-ASSISTED SINGLE-ARM PUSHUP

With these Pushups, one arm at a time does 70 percent or more of the work. The best place to start is with Staggered Pushups. The hand of the working arm should be placed flat on the floor underneath your shoulder.

The only difference is that you place the fingertips of your assisting arm on the floor. This puts the assisting hand in a weaker position, which shifts more of the weight onto your working arm.

Another option is the Uneven Pushup, where you place the hand of your assisting arm on an elevated surface like a low step, phone book, or basketball. The higher the surface, the less help the assisting arm can provide, making the exercise harder.

How to Do It

Starting Position

● Place the hand of your working arm flat on the floor underneath your shoulder.

● Place the fingertips of your assisting arm on the floor under your shoulder (a).

● Assume a hollow-body position: Squeeze your legs together, tense your thighs, glutes, and abs, and pull your ribs and shoulders down.

Perfect Execution

● Tuck your elbows to your sides and slowly pull yourself into the bottom position until your chest hovers just above the floor (b).

● Hold this bottom position briefly and squeeze your shoulder blades together.

● Then press through your armpits and reverse the movement, being sure to fully extend your arms, and push your shoulder blades away from each other at the top of the movement.

Your Goal

You should be able to perform multiple sets of 10 reps per side before moving to the next level.

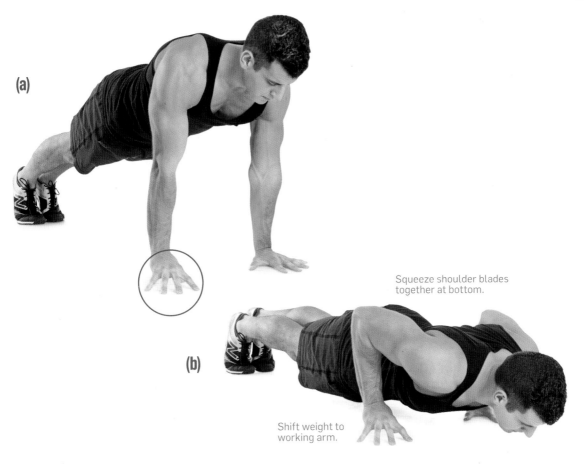

(a)

(b)

Squeeze shoulder blades together at bottom.

Shift weight to working arm.

Regressions

MAKE IT EASIER: Perform Eccentric Self-Assisted Single-Arm Pushups by doing only the lowering portion of the exercise (take at least 3 to 5 seconds to lower). Cheat into the top position by pushing up equally with both hands.

EVEN EASIER: Perform Isometric Self-Assisted Single-Arm Pushups by holding the bottom (or top) position.

EASIEST: Decrease the body angle by placing your hands on a sturdy box, bench, or chair. This makes it easier because you're pushing less body weight.

Progressions

MAKE IT HARDER: Use less self-assistance by placing fewer fingertips on the floor until only your thumb is touching the ground.

EVEN HARDER: Use less self-assistance and decrease your leverage with the Archer Pushup. Fully extend the arm of your assisting hand directly to the side, then perform a Pushup.

HARDEST: Increase the body angle by placing your feet on a sturdy box, bench, or chair. This makes it much harder because you're pushing more of your weight.

EVEN HARDER

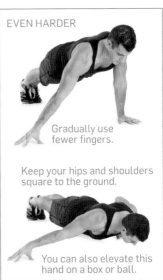

Gradually use fewer fingers.

Keep your hips and shoulders square to the ground.

You can also elevate this hand on a box or ball.

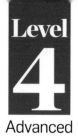
SINGLE-ARM PUSHUP

Studies show that you're pressing approximately 70 percent of your body weight during a floor Pushup. This means that a 200-pound man is pushing 140 pounds with every rep. Now if he can build up to doing Single-Arm Pushups for reps, it means he's pressing 140 pounds on one arm at a time. That's like repping out on Single-Arm Chest Presses with a 140-pound dumbbell!

When doing a Single-Arm Pushup, it is important to minimize body rotation and try to keep your hips and shoulders square to the floor. It's okay to rotate your nonworking shoulder and hip up and over toward your working arm as you lower to the bottom position in a diagonal fashion. However, you must do so with your hips and shoulders moving together with no twisting at the lower back. Your feet will also pivot a bit to allow for the hip rotation. This creates a criss-cross effect between your opposite shoulder and hip that makes the exercise easier to pull off.

How to Do It

Starting Position

- Place the hand of your working arm flat on the floor under your shoulder.
- Spread your fingers wide and grip the ground.
- Place your feet wider than shoulder-width apart for extra stability.
- Press the back of your nonworking hand into your lower back.
- Assume a hollow-body position: Tense your thighs, glutes, and abs, and pull your ribs and shoulders down.

Perfect Execution

- Tuck your elbow to your side and slowly pull yourself down until your chest hovers above the floor.
- Hold this bottom position briefly and squeeze the same-side shoulder blade in as if performing a Single-Arm Row.
- Then press through your armpit, being sure to fully extend your arm, and push your shoulder blade away at the top of the movement as if punching through the floor.

Your Goal

You should be able to perform multiple sets of 10 reps per side before moving to the next level.

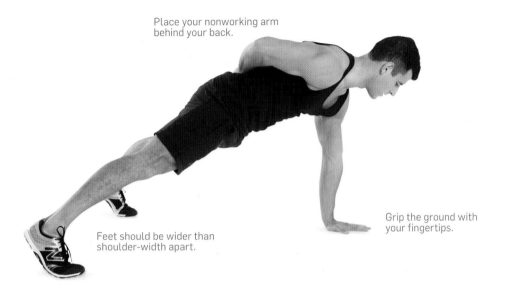

Place your nonworking arm behind your back.

Feet should be wider than shoulder-width apart.

Grip the ground with your fingertips.

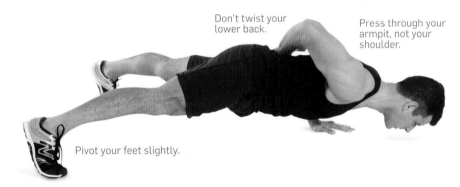

Don't twist your lower back.

Press through your armpit, not your shoulder.

Pivot your feet slightly.

Regressions

MAKE IT EASIER: Perform Eccentric Single-Arm Pushups by doing only the lowering portion of the exercise (take at least 3 to 5 seconds to lower). Cheat back up by pushing up with both hands.

EVEN EASIER: Perform Isometric Single-Arm Pushups by holding the bottom position. If you fatigue before time is up, simply back off to holding the top of the Pushup position.

EASIEST: Place your hands on a sturdy box, bench, or chair. This makes it much easier because you're pushing less of your body weight. Gradually work your way down to the floor over time by progressively decreasing the elevation height.

Progressions

MAKE IT HARDER: Perform Single-Arm, Single-Leg Pushups by raising the same-side leg as your working arm. Having only two points of contact with the ground amps up the abdominal work.

EVEN HARDER: Progressively bring your feet closer together until your feet are touching. This is the hardest version to do on the floor because it requires you to perform a Single-Arm Pushup with minimal to no hip and upper-back rotation.

HARDEST: Increase the body angle by performing Feet-Elevated Single-Arm Pushups. Place your feet on a sturdy box, bench, or chair.

PLYOMETRIC PUSHUP

Almost anybody can do a Plyo Pushup with his hands elevated on a bed or any other surface higher than waist height. That being said, it's important to prioritize strength and stability before adding speed and power into the equation. It will both build up the muscle you need to create force and move fast and prepare your joints and connective tissues for the rigors of explosive movement.

Start by holding the bottom Pushup position for 5 seconds before pushing off the ground with your hands. This will eliminate the stretch reflex, making your muscles work harder. You won't be able to get as much height, but it will groove great technique. And when you eventually perform fast reps with no pause at the bottom, you'll get some serious height. Also, treat each Plyo Pushup as a separate rep with a full pause between reps. This means that you'll land softly into the bottom of the Pushup position after going airborne and then push back up to the top of the Pushup position to gather yourself for the next Plyo Pushup. Never land with your arms locked out or you'll destroy your elbows.

How to Do It

Starting Position
- Place your hands directly underneath your shoulders with arms fully extended.
- Keep your weight over the center of your hands.
- Spread your fingertips as wide as you can.
- Assume a hollow-body position: Squeeze your legs together, tense your thighs, glutes, and abs, and pull your ribs and shoulders down.

Perfect Execution
- Tuck your elbows tight to your sides and slowly pull yourself into the bottom position until your chest hovers just above the floor.
- Hold this position for 5 seconds and squeeze your shoulder blades together.
- Explosively press through your armpits, extend your arms, and push off the ground with your fingertips so your body goes airborne.
- Land softly into the bottom of the Pushup position with your arms bent to absorb the load.

Your Goal
You should be able to perform multiple sets of 10 reps with perfect form and technique.

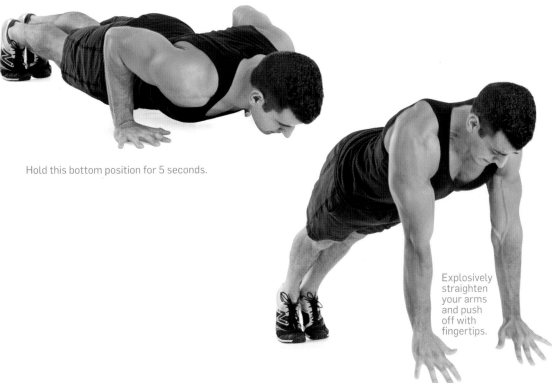

Hold this bottom position for 5 seconds.

Explosively straighten your arms and push off with fingertips.

Regressions

MAKE IT EASIER: Perform Drop Pushups. Start with your hands close together in the top of a Pushup position. Then jump your hands out to the sides and drop into the bottom position and repeat.

EVEN EASIER: Perform Speed Pushups by doing them as fast as you can while keeping your hands and feet on the floor.

EASIEST: Decrease the body angle by performing Hands-Elevated Plyo Pushups. Place your hands on a sturdy box, bench, or chair and do Explosive Pushups. This makes it much easier because you're pushing less of your body weight.

Progressions

MAKE IT HARDER: Perform Levitating Pushups where both your hands and feet leave the floor. Push off the floor with your toes and fingertips equally.

EVEN HARDER: Add a clap or multiple claps while airborne. You can also touch different parts of your body with your hands like your chest, shoulders, forehead, or even your hips. A favorite option is the Superman Pushup, where you fully extend your arms in front of your body while airborne.

HARDEST: Perform Feet-Elevated Plyo Pushups. Place your feet on a sturdy box or bench. This makes it much harder because you're pushing more of your body weight.

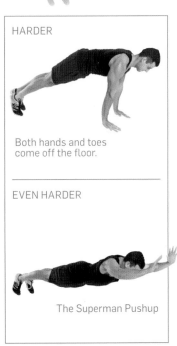

HARDER

Both hands and toes come off the floor.

EVEN HARDER

The Superman Pushup

Variations

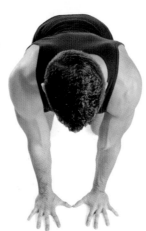

WIDE

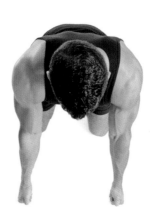

NARROW

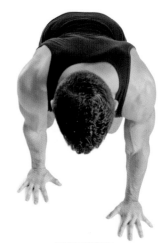

STAGGERED

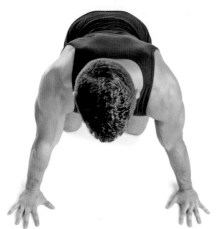

FINGERTIPS

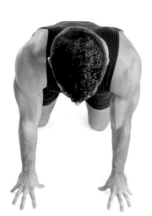

FISTS

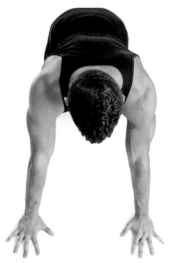

HIGH

1. Varying Hand Placement

Work your muscles from different angles by placing hands wider than shoulder-width apart, with thumbs touching and hands staggered. Placing your hands higher than shoulder level works your abs and triceps harder; hands lower (not shown) works the shoulders and chest more. Fingertip and Fist Pushups improve grip and wrist strength.

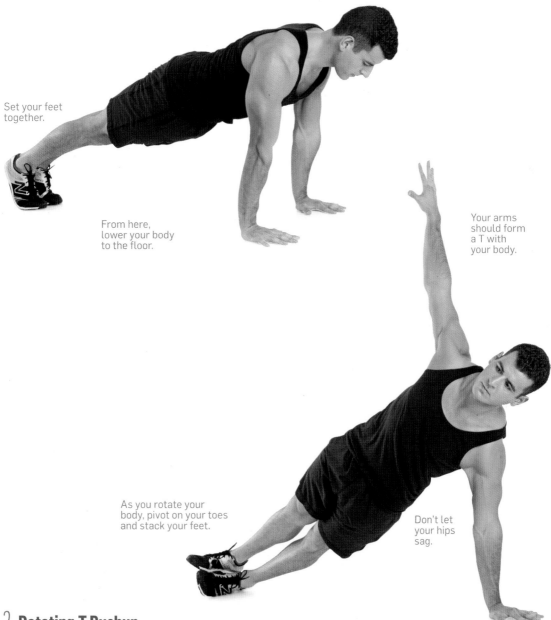

Set your feet together.

From here, lower your body to the floor.

Your arms should form a T with your body.

As you rotate your body, pivot on your toes and stack your feet.

Don't let your hips sag.

2. Rotating-T Pushup

Perform a Pushup and as you push yourself back up, rotate your body into a Side Plank so your right hand comes off the floor. Raise your right hand toward the ceiling so your body forms a T. Reverse the movement, switch sides, and repeat. If you can't perform the Pushup, simply hold the top of the Pushup position for a count before moving from side to side.

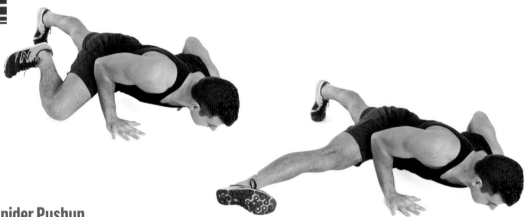

3. Spider Pushup

Flex your hip and bring one knee to the same-side elbow as you lower to the bottom position. You can make it even harder by fully extending that same leg to the side in the bottom position. This shifts more weight to the opposite arm for counterbalance. You can either perform all reps on one side before switching or switch sides every rep.

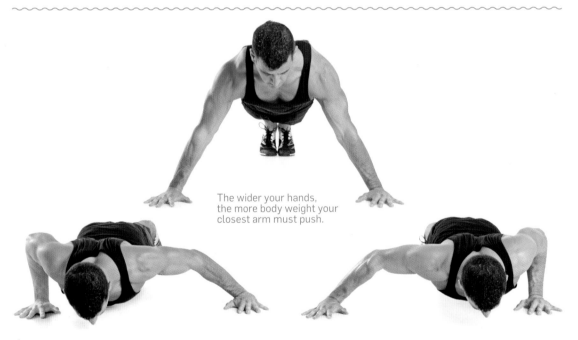

The wider your hands, the more body weight your closest arm must push.

4. Side-to-Side Pushup

Begin this exercise like a normal Wide-Hands Pushup, but as you lower your body to the ground, slowly shift your weight as much to one side as you can. Then push back up to the starting position. Switch sides every rep or perform all of your reps on one side before switching.

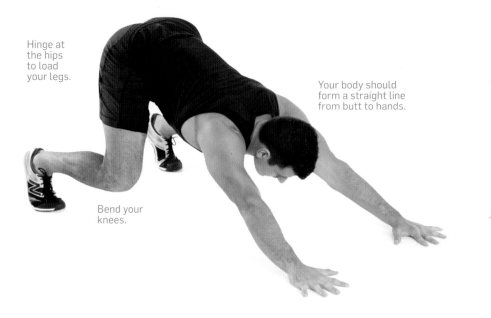

Hinge at the hips to load your legs.

Your body should form a straight line from butt to hands.

Bend your knees.

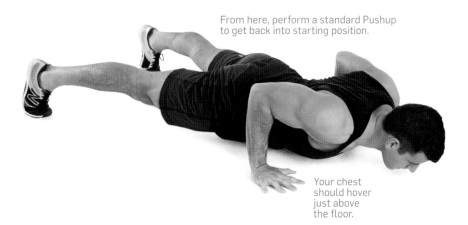

From here, perform a standard Pushup to get back into starting position.

Your chest should hover just above the floor.

5. Blast-Off Pushup

From the top of a standard Pushup position, push your butt back as far as you can by bending at the knees, hinging at the hips, and fully extending your arms. This is the loaded position. Now fire out by extending your ankles, knees, and hips into the bottom of a regular Pushup. Progress further by performing the move with your hands and feet closer together. You can also rock this drill with your feet against a wall to allow your legs to have better leverage to load and explode your body forward. This exercise improves ballistic core stability.

Chapter 7

BODYWEIGHT 8: DEEP SQUAT

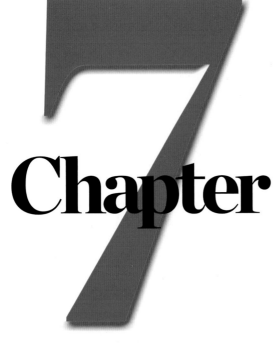

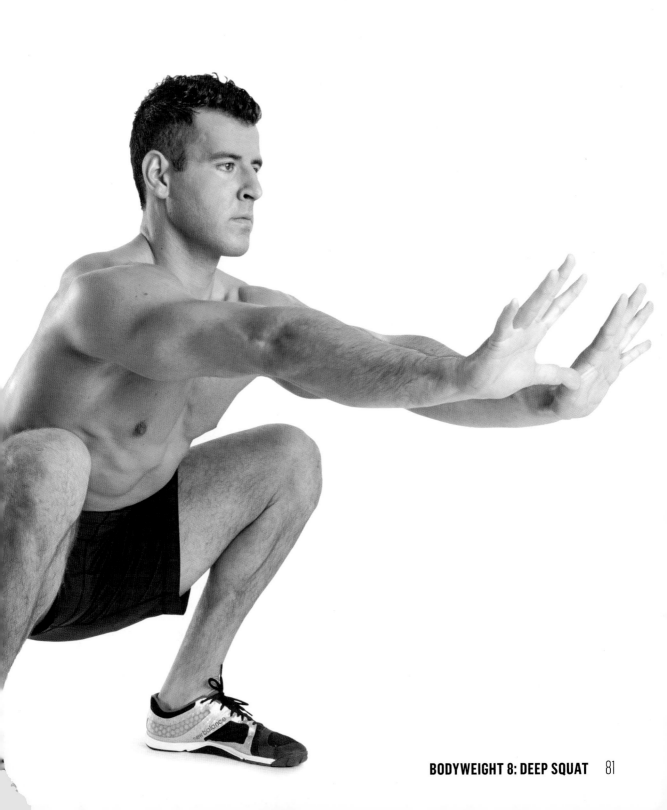

#3
DEEP SQUAT

The Deep Squat is the foundation of lower-body moves and may be the most important exercise you can do simply because it is such a functional movement. You squat every day of your life, and not just when you sit on the toilet. The way you squat dictates the way you do just about everything—sit down, stand up, walk, step, lunge, run, and jump—so you'd better do it right!

In many parts of the world, a Deep Squat is actually a position of rest, but in our tech-driven, sedentary American society, that couldn't be further from the truth. If you work at a desk, the deepest you'll squat all day is most likely determined by the depth of your chair. That's why most people have no idea what it means to perform a true Deep Squat. It doesn't mean your thighs are parallel to the floor. That's wrong. In a Deep Squat, you sit with your hamstrings resting on top of your calves and without overly rounding your lower back. To do it correctly requires a lot of core stability and mobility at your ankles, hips, and upper back. A Deep Squat requires full bending of your knees, something that many of us are unable to do without pain or discomfort. Years of not being in a Deep Squat will lead to an accumulation of soft-tissue restrictions all around your knees and even stiffness inside the joint capsule itself. It's no wonder so many people have achy, arthritic knees. To get the most out of bodyweight squatting, slow it down and focus less on reps and more on improving your range of motion.

Our goal in this chapter is to gradually achieve an ass-to-the-grass squat that brings a smile to your face (and to the faces of gawking strangers) every time you drop it like it's hot. Your knees and lower back will end up being so supple that you'll be able to sit in a Deep Squat for 5 to 10 minutes at a time without breaking a sweat. If you don't care about feeling and moving better, know this: Being a killer squatter is the quickest way to start looking hotter. Let's get to work!

The DEEP SQUAT Progression

Level 1	Level 2	Level 3	Level 4	Level 5
Ground Zero	Beginner	Intermediate	Advanced	Superhero
WALL SIT	BOX SQUAT	DEEP SQUAT	DEEP OVERHEAD SQUAT	JUMP SQUAT

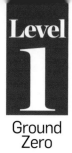

WALL SIT

The Wall Sit is an exercise that anybody can do, especially when modifying the range of motion by raising the hips above knee level as much as needed. It's a real safe, stable, and low-skill way to set up in a Squat position with perfect posture and to build strength. The upright and vertical trunk position shifts a greater emphasis to your quads (front thighs), helping you build up all of the muscles surrounding your knee to ensure that your patella (kneecap) tracks properly. This is especially important for people with a history of knee pain. Isometric holds like this are also easier on your joints than dynamic full-range-of-motion repetitions. Though this move is categorized as an entry-level exercise, it can continue to be used by more advanced trainees for warmups, active recovery, or endurance work. Plus, if you sink low enough so that your hips are below knee level, this move will challenge even the most fit amongst us. If you can't access a wall, simply use any flat and stable surface that's perpendicular to the floor, like a door or a pole.

How to Do It

Starting Position

- Stand in front of a wall with your feet hip- to shoulder-width apart.

- Establish tripod foot position for a natural foot arch.

- Raise your arms in front of you.

- Your toes should be pointing directly ahead, though a slight 10- to 20-degree toes-out position is acceptable, if needed.

Perfect Execution

- Sit into a Squat position with the tops of your front thighs parallel to the floor and your hips, upper back, and head in full contact with the wall.

- Sit as tall as possible and hold this position for time.

- If you fatigue before time is up, simply decrease the range of motion as much as needed midset to keep going.

Your Goal

You should be able to hold a Wall Sit for several 60-second sets with your hips below knee level before moving to the next level.

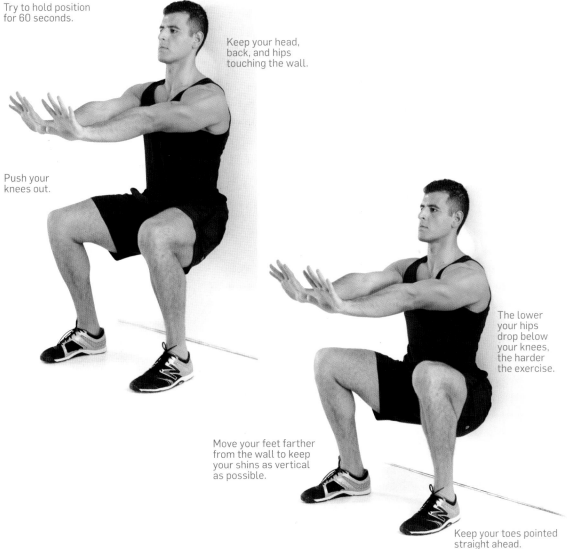

Try to hold position for 60 seconds.

Keep your head, back, and hips touching the wall.

Push your knees out.

The lower your hips drop below your knees, the harder the exercise.

Move your feet farther from the wall to keep your shins as vertical as possible.

Keep your toes pointed straight ahead.

Regressions

MAKE IT EASIER: Only lower to the point where your knees are bent at a 60- to 75-degree angle.

EVEN EASIER: Only lower to the point where your knees are bent at a 30- to 45-degree angle.

EASIEST: Only lower to the point where your knees are bent at a 10- to 15-degree angle.

Progressions

MAKE IT HARDER: Increase the range of motion so that your hips are lower than knee level.

EVEN HARDER: Move your feet closer together until they are touching.

HARDEST: Cross your arms with your hands resting on your shoulders (or hold your hands at chest level in prayer position). From there, place your hands behind your head (prisoner position) or extend your arms overhead.

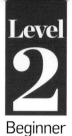
BOX SQUAT

The Box Squat is like training wheels for your bike. It allows you to build confidence and gradually prepare for the real thing without fear of falling. It's also a move you need to nail every time you sit down and stand up from a seated position. Sitting on a box has a built-in autocorrect feature that instantly fixes your form by making you bend at your hips before you bend at your knees as you aim for the target with your butt. That's the perfect form for doing a Squat. In doing so, it engrains the critical concept of keeping your shins as vertical as possible when squatting to save your knees. It also allows you to seamlessly scale the level of difficulty by increasing or decreasing the height of the box. For all of these reasons, the Box Squat should be a staple of your lower-body training, no matter how fit you are. It will also serve as a great tool to prepare you for Single-Leg Squats in Chapter 11.

How to Do It

Starting Position

● Assume tripod foot position with feet hip- to shoulder-width apart and heels placed in front of a sturdy box, step, bench, or ottoman. When seated, the tops of your thighs should be parallel to the floor.

● Your toes should point directly ahead, though a slight toes-out angle is acceptable.

● Assume a hollow-body position: Tense your thighs, glutes, and abs, and push your ribs and shoulders down.

Perfect Execution

● Push your hips and hamstrings back as far as you can (as if closing a door with your butt).

● Once your hips are fully stretched and loaded, bend at the knees, and slowly sit on the step.

● Briefly pause in the seated position while maintaining tension throughout your body, then hinge forward at your hips and stand up, squeezing your glutes.

Your Goal

You should be able to perform multiple sets of 10 reps before moving to the next level.

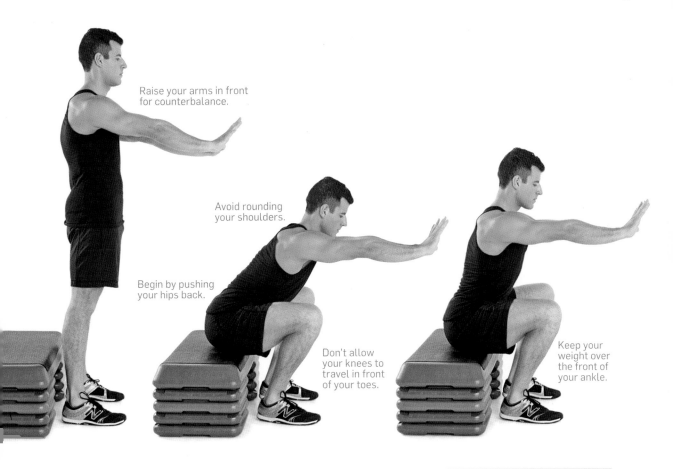

Raise your arms in front for counterbalance.

Avoid rounding your shoulders.

Begin by pushing your hips back.

Don't allow your knees to travel in front of your toes.

Keep your weight over the front of your ankle.

Regressions

MAKE IT EASIER: Decrease the range of motion by raising the height of the box so that your hips are slightly higher than your knees when seated.

EVEN EASIER: Raise the box even more.

EASIEST: Perform Self-Assisted Box Squats by holding a TRX (or another suspension trainer) or a stable support like a pole, railing, or ledge. This will allow you to use as much upper-body assistance as necessary to perform the movement pain-free through a full range of motion.

Progressions

MAKE IT HARDER: Increase the range of motion by lowering the height of the box so that your hips are slightly lower than your knees when seated.

EVEN HARDER: Lower the box even more.

HARDEST: Perform a Deep Box Squat by lowering the height of the box so much that your hamstrings rest on your calves when seated. This is the exact range of motion you'll need for Deep Squats without a box.

Tool Tip

Use an aerobics step with adjustable risers because it allows you to seamlessly adjust the height of the box a couple inches at a time. It's particularly useful for the Deep Box Squat because it can be adjusted very low so you're just above the floor while seated. If you don't have an adjustable step, any stable box, chair, bench, or ottoman will work.

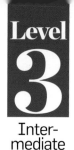

DEEP SQUAT

The beauty of bodyweight training is that you can forget about adding weight plates and simply focus on increasing range of motion an inch at a time. Progressing gradually will unlock your full potential and protect your knees and back. Initially, limit your depth to the point where you start to round your lower back. Your first goal is to be able to squat low enough so that the tops of your front thighs are parallel to the floor with your hips and knees on the same level (a). The next step is to achieve a depth where your hips are lower than your knees. The final step is to be able to sink super low so that your hamstrings rest on your calves (b). Take your time and be patient, because achieving the Deep Squat position is one of the most important standards.

At a certain depth, your knees will inch forward as your ankles bend more. This ankle bend makes your calves and shins work harder. Just be aware of keeping your shins as vertical as possible to avoid injury.

How to Do It

Starting Position

• Assume tripod foot position with your feet hip- to shoulder-width apart. Your toes should be pointing directly ahead, though a slight toes-out position is acceptable.

• Set your head in a neutral position with ears aligned with your shoulders, hips, and ankles, and keep your gaze ahead.

• Assume a hollow-body position: Tense your thighs, glutes, and abs, and push your ribs and shoulders down.

Perfect Execution

• First, push your hips and hamstrings back as far as you can (as if closing a door with your butt).

• Once your hips are fully stretched and loaded, bend at the knees, and slowly squat. Go as low as you can without overly rounding your lower back.

• Pause in the bottom position while maintaining tension throughout your body, then stand, squeezing your glutes.

Your Goal

You should be able to perform multiple sets of 10 reps before moving to the next level.

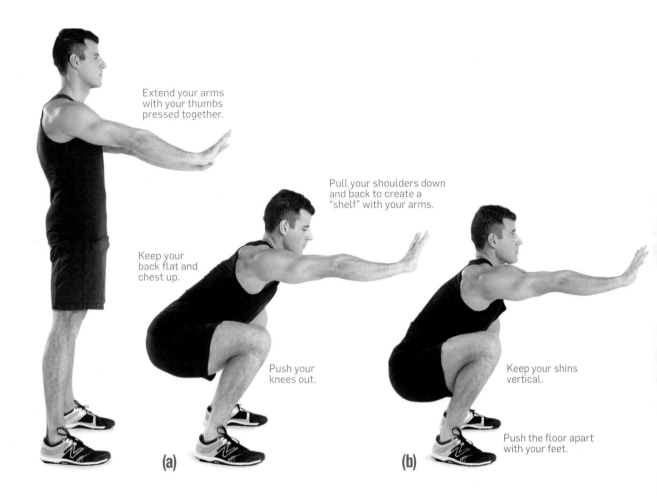

Extend your arms with your thumbs pressed together.

Pull your shoulders down and back to create a "shelf" with your arms.

Keep your back flat and chest up.

Push your knees out.

Keep your shins vertical.

Push the floor apart with your feet.

(a)

(b)

Regressions

MAKE IT EASIER: Decrease the range of motion by only squatting down to the point where the tops of your front thighs are parallel to the floor (a).

EVEN EASIER: Squat to the point where you can maintain a neutral spine position without knee pain.

EASIEST: Perform Self-Assisted Deep Squats by holding on to a suspension trainer or a stable support like a pole, railing, or ledge. This will allow you to use as much upper-body assistance as necessary to perform the move through a full range of motion.

Progressions

MAKE IT HARDER: Increase the range of motion by squatting down low enough so that your hips are lower than your knees.

EVEN HARDER: Squat until your hamstrings rest on your calves in the rock-bottom squatting position (b).

HARDEST: Further increase the range of motion by performing Close-Stance Deep Squats where your feet are only hip-width apart or narrower. This variation prepares you for the high ankle and hip mobility demands of a Deep Single-Leg Squat (aka Pistol Squat) while still using both legs.

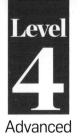

DEEP OVERHEAD SQUAT

By now, you've already gained the prerequisite mobility in your ankles, knees, and hips, but extending your arms overhead is a game-changer. Most people hyperextend their lower back and allow their ribs to rise when reaching overhead, putting their back and shoulders in compromised positions. You need to brace your core, get your ribs and shoulders down, and have a lot of mobility at your thoracic spine. Sink to a depth that allows you to maintain this safe neutral spine position.

Hunching over a computer all day leads to tight muscles in your chest, lats, and shoulders that make it very difficult to fully extend your arms overhead properly. So, try this trick: Hold on to a resistance band, towel, or rope. Don't just hold it— actively try to pull it apart and break it (don't worry, you won't). This will make it easier to maintain the overhead-arms positioning because it stabilizes your shoulders and activates your upper-back muscles.

How to Do It

Starting Position

• Assume tripod foot position with your feet hip-to shoulder-width apart. Your toes should be pointing directly ahead, though a slight toes-out position is acceptable.

• Assume a hollow-body position: Tense your thighs, glutes, and abs, and push your ribs and shoulders down.

• Extend your arms overhead without allowing your lower back to hyperextend.

Perfect Execution

• First, push your hips and hamstrings back as far as you can (as if closing a door with your butt).

• Once your hips are fully stretched and loaded, bend at the knees, and squat. Go as low as you can without overly rounding your lower back.

• Pause in the bottom position while maintaining tension throughout your body, then stand, squeezing your glutes.

Your Goal

You should be able to perform multiple sets of 10 reps before moving to the next level.

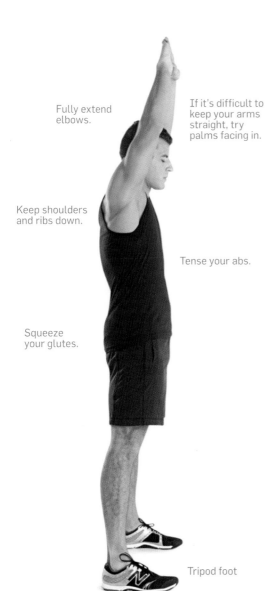

Fully extend elbows.

If it's difficult to keep your arms straight, try palms facing in.

Keep shoulders and ribs down.

Tense your abs.

Squeeze your glutes.

Tripod foot

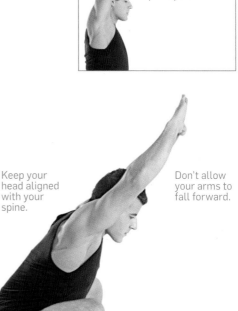

To stabilize shoulders, hold a towel between hands and pull apart.

Keep your head aligned with your spine.

Don't allow your arms to fall forward.

Regressions

MAKE IT EASIER: Sit on a low box so that your hamstrings rest on your calves.

EVEN EASIER: Perform a Deep Prisoner Squat by interlocking your hands behind your head while squeezing your shoulder blades together.

EASIEST: Perform a Deep Prayer Squat with your hands together at chest level as if praying.

Progressions

MAKE IT HARDER: Bring your hands closer together until ideally they are touching. It will be easier to stabilize your shoulders with your palms facing each other.

EVEN HARDER: Bring your feet closer together until they are touching.

HARDEST: Bring both your hands and feet closer together until they are touching.

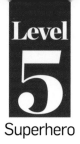

JUMP SQUAT

Now that you've nailed flawless deep squatting, it's time to add power to those legs. Add explosive movement by jumping out of the bottom of a Squat and going airborne. Anytime your feet leave the floor, it becomes much harder to reestablish tripod foot position, keep your shins vertical, and get your knees out when landing into the Squat position.

To master it, lower only to the point where the tops of your front thighs are parallel to the floor. Pause and hold this bottom position for 5 seconds. This will eliminate the stretch reflex, making your muscles work harder while taking pressure off your joints and connective tissues. Eventually, you can progress to performing continuous Jump Squats without a pause at the bottom. Partial Jump Squats aren't just a regression. If you look at most explosive actions in sports, they take place with minimal bending at the knees and hips. So Partial Jump Squats, with your hips above knee level, are a viable exercise option to use in your training program.

How to Do It

Starting Position

- Assume tripod foot position with your feet hip- to shoulder-width apart. Your toes should be pointing directly ahead or slightly outward.

- Set your head in a neutral position and extend your arms in front of you.

- Assume a hollow-body position: Tense your thighs, clench your glutes, brace your abs, and push your ribs and shoulders down.

Perfect Execution

- First, push your hips and hamstrings back as far as you can (as if closing a door with your butt).

- Once your hips are fully stretched and loaded, bend at the knees, and then slowly squat into the bottom position with the tops of your thighs parallel to the floor.

- Pause for 5 seconds in the bottom position, and then jump as high as you can, landing softly into the bottom position.

Your Goal

You should be able to do multiple sets of 10 perfect reps with a lot of height on each jump and super-soft landings.

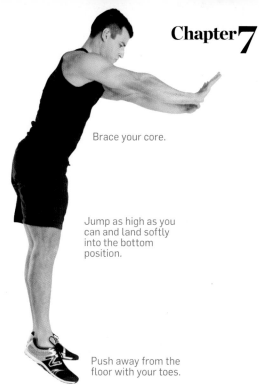

Brace your core.

Jump as high as you can and land softly into the bottom position.

Push away from the floor with your toes.

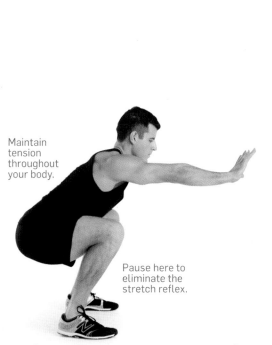

Maintain tension throughout your body.

Pause here to eliminate the stretch reflex.

Regressions

MAKE IT EASIER: Perform Partial Jump Squats by squatting only to the point where you can maintain a neutral spine position without knee pain.

EVEN EASIER: Jump off a box or bench from a Squat position and then land softly into that same position. Not only does this move autocorrect your form, but it is lower impact and it also builds starting strength because you are exploding out of a dead-stop position.

EASIEST: Perform Self-Assisted Jump Squats by holding a suspension trainer or a pole, railing, or ledge. This will allow you to use as much assistance as necessary to perform the move pain-free through a full range of motion.

Progressions

MAKE IT HARDER: Squat low enough so that your hips are beneath your knees. If you go all the way down into the bottom of the Deep Squat position with your hamstrings resting on your calves, be sure you don't bounce, as that can put undue strain on your knees. Rather, pause and hold this deep position briefly before exploding back up.

EVEN HARDER: Jump from a staggered stance position with the toes of one leg aligned with the heel of your other leg. Perform all of your reps on the same side before switching or switch legs midair every rep.

HARDEST: Jump from a split stance or the bottom of a Lunge. The foot of your leading leg should be flat, and you should be on the toes of your trailing leg. Perform all of your reps on the same side before switching or switch legs midair every rep.

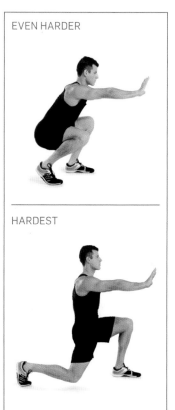

EVEN HARDER

HARDEST

Variations

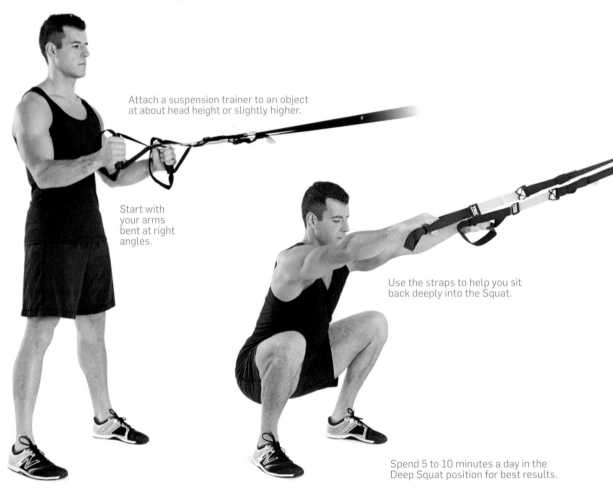

Attach a suspension trainer to an object at about head height or slightly higher.

Start with your arms bent at right angles.

Use the straps to help you sit back deeply into the Squat.

Spend 5 to 10 minutes a day in the Deep Squat position for best results.

1. TRX-Assisted Deep Squat

Attach a TRX strap or other suspension trainer to a sturdy object. Grasp the handles and walk backward until it's taut. Hold the handles at chest height with your elbows bent 90 degrees. With feet about shoulder-width apart, perform a Deep Squat by sitting back at the hips and bending your legs. Allow your arms to straighten if needed. Pull on the straps for as much assistance as you need going down and pushing back up to perform the Deep Squat with flawless form.

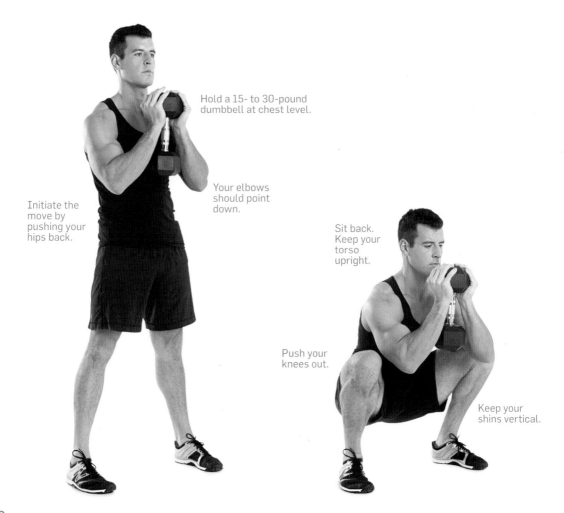

Hold a 15- to 30-pound dumbbell at chest level.

Your elbows should point down.

Initiate the move by pushing your hips back.

Sit back. Keep your torso upright.

Push your knees out.

Keep your shins vertical.

2. Goblet Squat

Sometimes adding weight to an exercise actually makes it easier. In this case, holding on to a weight at chest level provides counterbalance that allows you to sit your hips back more without the fear of falling backward. It also allows you to keep your trunk more upright and sink into a deeper Squat. This move can be performed by holding a dumbbell, kettlebell, or even a medicine ball or sandbag. Either hold a vertically oriented dumbbell with your hands clasped underneath the top end or hold a kettlebell by the horns or squeeze a heavier bag or ball between your hands. Keep the weight at chest level, with your elbows up and tight to your sides.

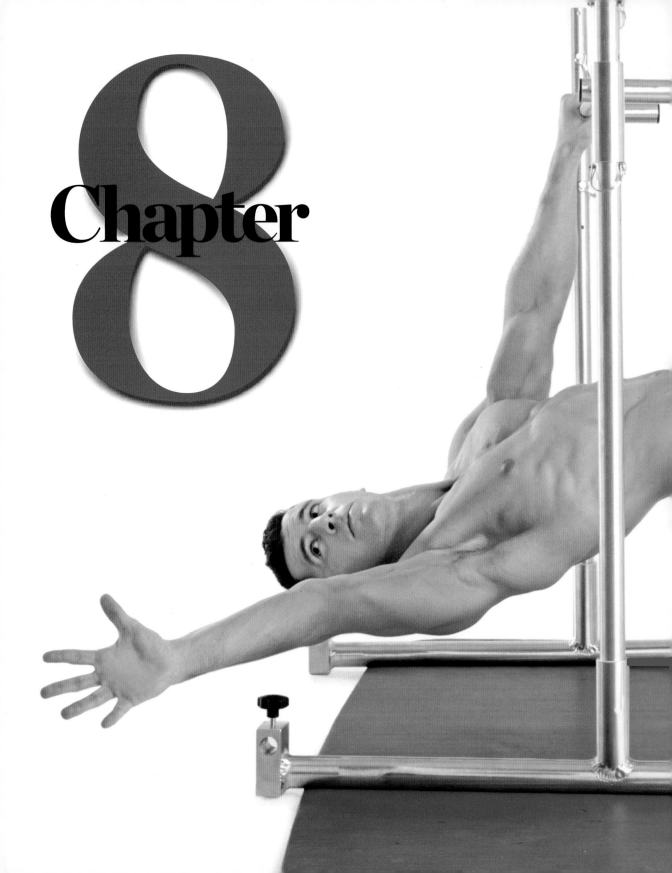

Chapter 8

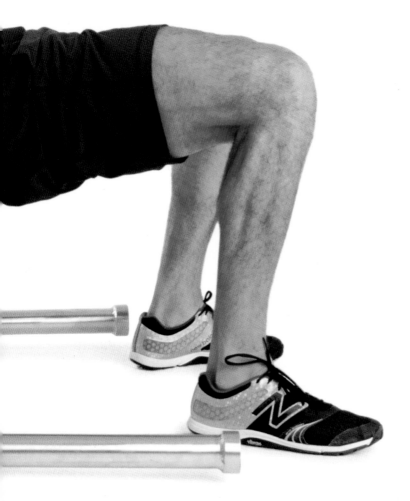

BODYWEIGHT 8: ROW

#4 ROW

The Row is the best exercise to build your entire back side. Pulling your body up works your biceps, forearms, lats, upper back/midback, traps, and rear shoulders. In addition, because you're pulling your body in a horizontal position, your lower back, glutes, and hamstrings have to work hard to keep your body in a rigid Plank position. Even your abs have to kick in to stabilize your spine so that you don't hyperextend your lower back. The Row is also easier to perform than a Pullup because you're pulling less of your total body weight.

The bodyweight Row offers advantages over the barbell Bent-Over Row: One, the bodyweight Row doesn't require as much hamstring flexibility and lower-back strength as pulling a heavy barbell from a hip-hinged position. Two, the bodyweight Row allows you to quickly adjust your body angle and foot position to make the exercise easier or harder as needed. With a barbell Row, you have to set the bar down and then add or subtract weight. Three, the bodyweight Row is the exact opposite movement pattern as the Pushup. The better you get at Rows, the better you will get at Pushups. The Row is the first bodyweight exercise in this book that requires equipment of some kind. After all, you can't really pull yourself unless you have something to hold on to. The best options are a Pullup bar that's set at about hip height or a TRX (or another suspension trainer) that you can anchor to a door, wall, ceiling, pole, or tree. If you don't want to spend money on equipment, here are some alternatives perfect for rowing at home or in a hotel room.

❶ Place your body underneath a sturdy table and hold on to the table sides with your palms facing each other, or the bottom end of the table with an underhand grip, or the top end of the table with an overhand grip. If you have a long enough towel, you can wrap it around the table and hold one end in each hand.

❷ Hold on to a horizontal pole or railing with both hands or grip a vertical pole, ledge, or tree like a baseball bat. The towel-wrapping technique works here, too.

❸ Grab each edge of a door frame with the same-side hand with your palms facing away from your body. Or grab a single edge of the door frame with the fingertips of both hands, which really challenges your grip.

❹ Hold on to the seats of two sturdy chairs that are ideally hip height off the floor.

❺ Place a thick broomstick over the tops of two boxes or chairs of even height to serve as your rowing bar.

The ROW Progression

Level 1	Level 2	Level 3	Level 4	Level 5
Ground Zero	Beginner	Intermediate	Advanced	Superhero
HANGING BRIDGE	ROW	SELF-ASSISTED SINGLE-ARM ROW	SINGLE-ARM ROW	PLYOMETRIC ROW

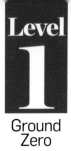
HANGING BRIDGE

The Hanging Bridge is to the Row as the Plank is to the Pushup. It sets the foundation for all the progressions to follow by teaching you how to hold the start with a hollow-body position. Use a hook grip as much as possible. Wrap your fingers over the top of the bar and your thumb under the bar. From there, try to clasp your thumb around your index and/or middle finger. Flex your wrists slightly so that your pinkie finger will slide over the top of the bar. This is your strongest gripping position. It puts your shoulders into the most stable position because it creates an external rotation force that screws them into their sockets. If the bar is too thick to use a hook grip, wrap all five digits over the top of the bar and press your thumb into your index finger to lock in.

FOOT PLACEMENT: Keep your feet together. Though technically this provides you with a smaller base of support than a wider foot placement, it makes it much easier to engage your hip and core muscles to maintain a neutral spine position with a slight arch in your lower back.

How to Do It

Starting Position

● Grab the bar or handles of a suspension trainer with a hook grip.

● Set your head in a neutral position with your ears aligned with your shoulders, hips, and ankles, and look between your hands.

● With legs fully extended in front of your body and your heels on the floor, lift your hips until your body forms a straight line from your head through heels.

● Assume a hollow-body position with your toes pointing up. Squeeze your legs together, tense your thighs, glutes, and abs, and pull your ribs and shoulders down.

Perfect Execution

● Hold this Hanging Bridge position for time while actively maintaining hollow-body form for the duration of the exercise.

● Focus on deep belly breathing to prevent your ribs from rising.

Your Goal

You should be able to do multiple sets of 60-second holds before moving to the next level.

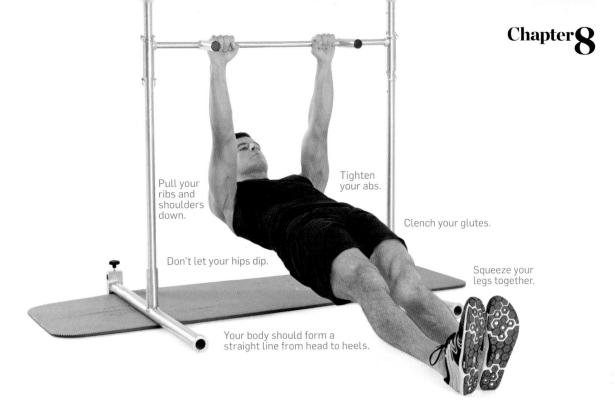

Pull your ribs and shoulders down.

Tighten your abs.

Clench your glutes.

Don't let your hips dip.

Squeeze your legs together.

Your body should form a straight line from head to heels.

Regressions

MAKE IT EASIER: Increase your base of support by widening your hands or your feet.

EVEN EASIER: Bend your knees and place your feet directly underneath your knees.

EASIEST: Decrease your body angle by performing an Inclined Hanging Bridge. This is easier because you're holding less of your body weight. This will work best while holding on to a pole, railing, or door frame or by using a TRX suspension trainer. These gripping options allow you to walk your feet forward and backward to make the move harder or easier as needed.

Progressions

MAKE IT HARDER: Use a narrower grip. Progressively bring your hands closer together until your thumbs are touching.

EVEN HARDER: Perform a Feet-Elevated Hanging Bridge by putting your feet on a sturdy box or bench.

HARDEST: Perform a Single-Leg Hanging Bridge. Lift one leg off the floor and focus on squeezing the glute of your supporting leg to keep your hips square to the ground (a). Further decrease stability by performing a Single-Arm Hanging Bridge. Place the hand of your working arm directly underneath your same-side shoulder, your feet shoulder-width apart for balance, and then take one hand off of the bar (b). Feeling strong? Next, raise the leg opposite your nonworking arm (c).

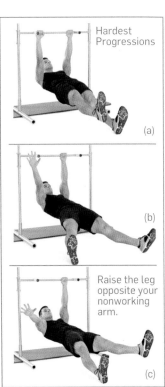

Hardest Progressions

(a)

(b)

Raise the leg opposite your nonworking arm.

(c)

ROW

The Row is the exact opposite movement pattern of the Pushup, making it a perfect exercise to superset or alternate between. Rows require you to keep your forearms as vertical as possible. This will save your elbows. A good rule of thumb is to perform at least as many total sets and reps for Rows as you do for Pushups. If you have shoulder pain or do lots of bench-pressing with very few pulling exercises, then do two to three times the sets or reps of Rows as you do of Pushups to correct this structural imbalance.

There are many grips you can use. A normal grip is overhand, about shoulder-width apart. You can go wider to make your upper back and rear shoulders work harder or closer to make your forearms and biceps work harder. Use an under-hand grip to shift the work more to your biceps. If you're holding on to a set of parallel bars, the sides of a sturdy table, or even the outsides of two chairs of equal height, then you can perform Rows with a neutral grip with palms facing each other. Using a TRX (or another suspension trainer) allows you to rotate your hands as you pull, which tends to be easier on the shoulders.

How to Do It

Starting Position

- Grab the bar or handles of a suspension trainer with a hook grip.

- Set your head in a neutral position with your ears aligned with your shoulders, hips, and ankles, and look between your hands.

- With legs fully extended, lift your hips until your body forms a straight line from your head to heels.

- Assume a hollow-body position. Squeeze your legs together, tense your thighs, glutes, and abs, and pull your ribs and shoulders down.

Perfect Execution

- Initiate the movement by pulling your shoulders down and back and driving your elbows tight to your sides.

- When your elbows are bent at 90-degree angles, hold this position for 1 or 2 seconds and visualize trying to crack a walnut between your shoulder blades.

- Reverse the movement and repeat.

Your Goal

You should be able to do multiple sets of 10 reps before moving to the next level.

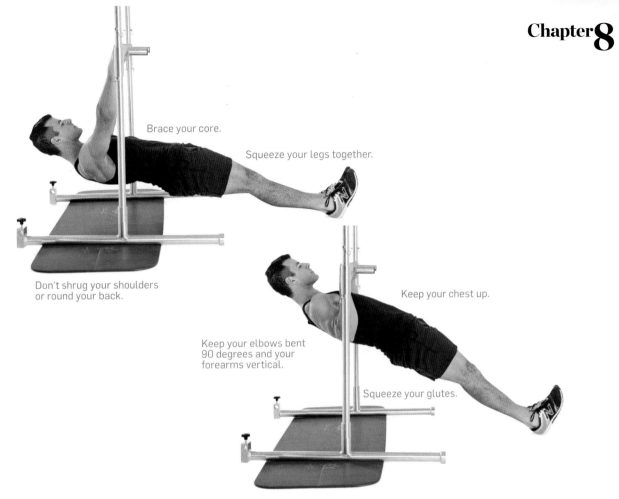

Brace your core.

Squeeze your legs together.

Don't shrug your shoulders or round your back.

Keep your chest up.

Keep your elbows bent 90 degrees and your forearms vertical.

Squeeze your glutes.

Regressions

MAKE IT EASIER: Increase your base of support by widening your hands or feet.

EVEN EASIER: Bend your legs and place your feet underneath your knees.

EASIEST: Decrease your body angle by performing an Inclined Row. Stand holding a pole, door frame, or the handles of a suspension trainer. These gripping options allow you to walk your feet forward or backward to change the incline of your body. Lean back until your arms are straight. This is the starting position. Now bend your arms to pull yourself forward and return. Repeat.

Progressions

MAKE IT HARDER: Progressively bring your hands closer together until your thumbs are touching.

EVEN HARDER: Lift one leg off the floor and squeeze the glute of your supporting leg to keep your hips square to the ground.

HARDEST: Increase the body angle by performing Feet-Elevated Rows (shown). Place your feet on a sturdy box. This forces you to pull more of your body weight. Make it super hard by elevating your feet above shoulder level.

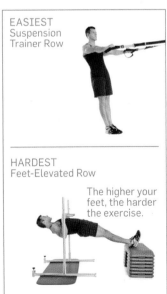

EASIEST Suspension Trainer Row

HARDEST Feet-Elevated Row

The higher your feet, the harder the exercise.

SELF-ASSISTED SINGLE-ARM ROW

With these Rows, one arm does about 70 percent of the work or more. One option is the Uneven Row. The hand of the working arm should grab the rowing bar as normal. The only difference is that you place a thick towel or rope around the bar and hold the ends of the towel in the assisting hand. The lower you grab on the towel, the greater the mechanical disadvantage to that arm—making it harder to assist and further challenging your working arm. I like this option because gripping a towel with your assisting hand works your grip in a more complete way, providing a greater challenge to your thumb and palm muscles.

How to Do It

Starting Position

- Grab the bar with your working arm just underneath your shoulder.

- Wrap a towel around the bar and grab both ends with your assisting hand.

- With your legs fully extended, place your feet on a bench.

- Assume a hollow-body position. Squeeze your legs together, tense your thighs, glutes, and abs, and pull your ribs and shoulders down.

Perfect Execution

- Initiate the movement by pulling your shoulders down and back and bending your elbows.

- Once you reach the point where your working-arm elbow is bent at 90 degrees, hold this position for 1 or 2 seconds and visualize trying to crack a walnut between your shoulder blades.

- Then reverse the movement and repeat.

Your Goal

You should be able to do multiple sets of 10 reps per side before moving to the next level.

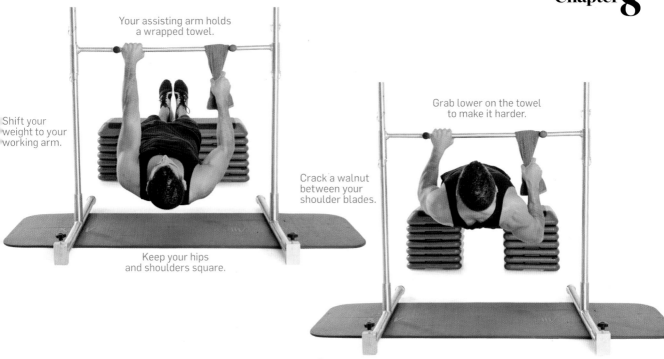

Your assisting arm holds a wrapped towel.

Shift your weight to your working arm.

Keep your hips and shoulders square.

Crack a walnut between your shoulder blades.

Grab lower on the towel to make it harder.

Regressions

MAKE IT EASIER: Increase your base of support by widening your feet.

EVEN EASIER: Improve your leverage by bending your legs and placing your feet directly underneath your knees.

EASIEST: Inclined Self-Assisted Single-Arm Rows. This is easier because it requires you to hold less of your body weight. This will work best while holding on to a pole, railing, or door frame or by using a suspension trainer. The gripping options allow you to seamlessly walk your feet forward and backward to make the move harder or easier as needed.

Progressions

MAKE IT HARDER: Use less assistance and decrease your leverage with the Archer Row. Fully extend the arm of your assisting hand directly to the side to force your working arm to bear the bulk of your weight. Complete all reps using this working arm before switching arm positions and repeating the exercise for your other arm.

EVEN HARDER: Perform an Archer Row but progressively use fewer fingers of the assisting hand on the bar until only one or two fingers remain.

HARDEST: Perform Single-Leg Self-Assisted Single-Arm Rows. Lift one leg off the bench and really focus on squeezing the glute of your supporting leg to keep your hips square to the ground. This variation will enhance the glute and hamstring work for your supporting leg.

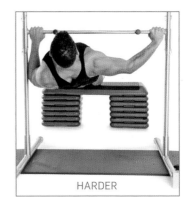

HARDER

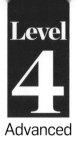
SINGLE-ARM ROW

In this move, if your abs, lower back, and hips don't work perfectly in concert, your body will twist and turn like you're getting down at a '70s disco. That's why unlike in the other levels, you should start with your legs bent and feet underneath your knees to make the task more manageable. It helps a great deal to reach your nonworking arm on the body side of the bar or past the handle as you pull up. This will provide some counterbalance.

Though you want to minimize body rotation and keep your hips and shoulders as square to the floor as possible, it's okay to rotate your trailing shoulder and hip up and over toward your working arm as you pull up into the top position in kind of a diagonal fashion. However, you must do so with your hips and shoulders moving together and with no twisting at the lower back.

How to Do It

Starting Position

- Using one hand, grab the bar with a hook grip. Extend your nonworking arm toward the ceiling.

- With your legs bent and your feet underneath your knees, lift your hips until they are fully extended and your body forms a straight line from your head to your knees.

- Place your feet wider than shoulder-width apart for extra stability.

- Assume a hollow-body position: Clench your glutes, brace your abs, and pull your ribs and shoulders down.

Perfect Execution

- Initiate the movement by pulling your shoulders down and back and driving your elbow tight to your side.

- Once you reach the point where your elbow is bent at a 90-degree angle, hold this position for 1 or 2 seconds and squeeze your shoulder blades together as if trying to crack a walnut between them.

- Then reverse the movement and repeat. Keep your hips fully extended throughout the movement.

Your Goal

You should be able to do multiple sets of 10 reps per side before moving to the next level.

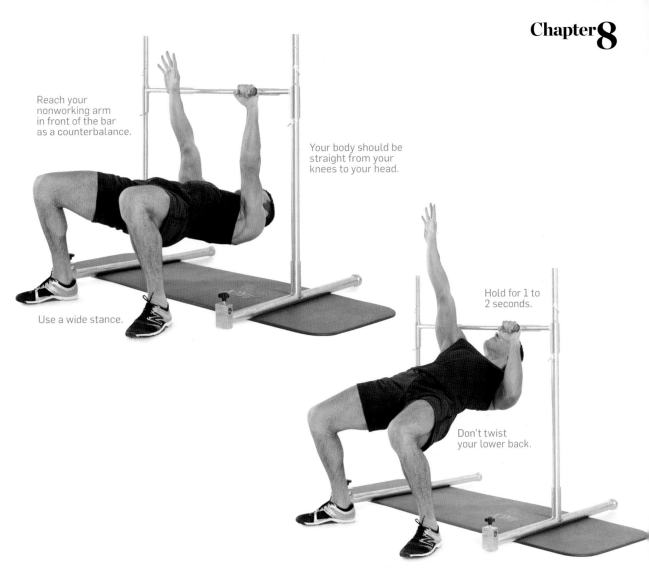

Reach your nonworking arm in front of the bar as a counterbalance.

Your body should be straight from your knees to your head.

Use a wide stance.

Hold for 1 to 2 seconds.

Don't twist your lower back.

Regressions

MAKE IT EASIER: Perform Eccentric Single-Arm Rows by only doing the lowering portion of the exercise (lower for at least 3 to 5 seconds) and then cheating back up into the top position by pulling up equally with both hands.

EVEN EASIER: Perform Isometric Single-Arm Rows by holding the top (or bottom) position.

EASIEST: Eliminate your body angle by performing Inclined Single-Arm Rows. This will work best while holding on to a pole or door frame or by using a TRX suspension trainer while standing straight. The gripping options allow you to walk your feet forward and backward to make the move harder or easier.

Progressions

MAKE IT HARDER: Decrease your base of support by bringing your feet closer together until they touch.

EVEN HARDER: Lift the same-side leg of your working arm off the floor and squeeze the glute of your supporting leg to keep your hips square to the ground.

HARDEST: Increase the relative loading by fully extending your legs straight out in front of your body. This makes it ultra difficult to keep your hips fully extended and requires you to pull more of your total body weight. Make it even harder by elevating your feet. If you can pull that off, you're crazy strong.

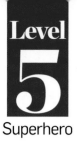

PLYOMETRIC ROW

One of the big knocks on bodyweight training is that it doesn't allow you to train explosive pulling power like you can with weights. Olympic lifting movements like Snatches, Cleans, and High Pulls or even kettlebell exercises like Swings allow you to transfer force from your lower body through your upper body by forcefully extending your ankles, knees, and hips and pulling a weight with your arms. The Plyometric Row is the body-weight answer. Start with your legs bent and your feet underneath your knees to make the task more manageable. Also hold the top of the rowing position for 5 seconds before each explosive rep to keep your form clean in the beginning. Later, you can progress to performing continuous reps without pausing.

How to Do It

Starting Position

- Grab the bar or handles of a suspension trainer with a hook grip.

- With your legs bent and your feet underneath your knees, lift your hips until they are fully extended and your body forms a straight line from your head through your knees.

- Assume a hollow-body position: Clench your glutes, brace your abs, and pull your ribs and shoulders down.

Perfect Execution

- Initiate the movement by pulling your shoulders down and back and driving your elbows tight to your sides.

- Once you reach the point where your elbows are bent at 90-degree angles, hold this position for 5 seconds and visualize trying to crack a walnut between your shoulder blades.

- Then quickly reverse the movement and lower your body to the starting position and then immediately pull right back up to the top position as fast as you can and repeat. You must keep your hips fully extended throughout the movement.

Your Goal

You should be able to do multiple sets of 10 reps.

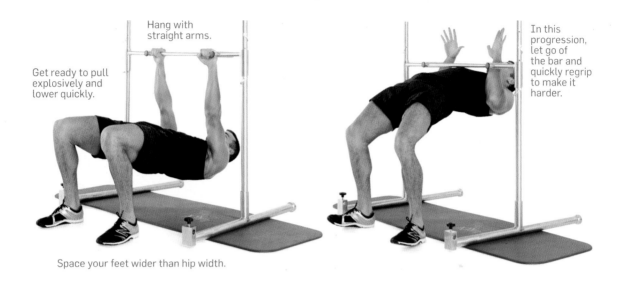

Get ready to pull explosively and lower quickly.

Hang with straight arms.

Space your feet wider than hip width.

In this progression, let go of the bar and quickly regrip to make it harder.

Regressions

MAKE IT EASIER: Hold the easier bottom position with your arms fully extended for 5 seconds.

EVEN EASIER: Perform Inclined Plyometric Rows. This will work best while holding on to a pole, railing, or by using a TRX suspension trainer. The gripping options allow you to walk your feet forward and backward to make the move harder or easier as needed.

EASIEST: Perform Jump Squat Rows. Integrate a Jump Squat with a Plyo Row for an unmatched total-body metabolic move. Assisting with your legs allows your arms to pull less weight and to be more explosive. This works best by holding on to a pole or, ideally, the handles of a suspension trainer that is anchored to a wall. Squat until your arms are fully extended and then simultaneously jump up and pull your hands to your armpits, going airborne. Land softly into the bottom of the Squat, pause, and repeat.

Progressions

MAKE IT HARDER: If you're holding on to a straight bar or two parallel bars, allow your hands to go airborne at the apex of every pull and then regrip as you begin your descent. Add a clap at the top or change your hand placement midair, alternating between a wider grip, normal grip, closer grip, or even a mixed grip with one hand overhand and the other underhand.

EVEN HARDER: Extend your legs straight out in front of your body. This makes it ultradifficult to keep your hips fully extended and requires you to pull more of your total body weight.

HARDEST: Increase the body angle by performing Feet-Elevated Plyo Rows. Place your feet on a stable box, bench, chair, or ottoman. Make it super hard by elevating your feet above shoulder level.

Variations

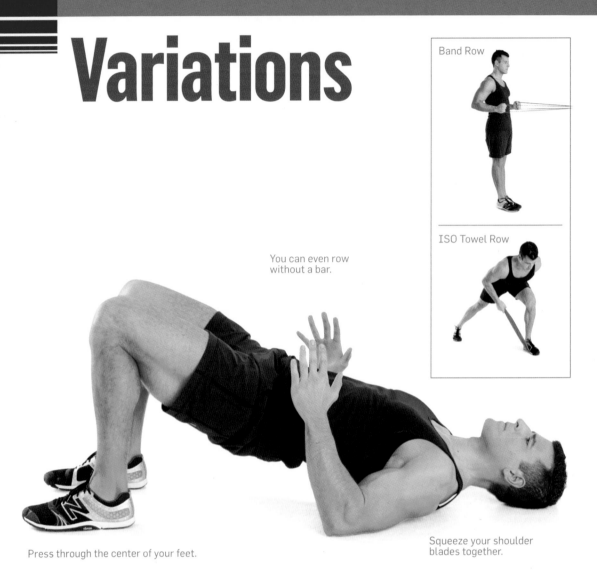

Band Row

ISO Towel Row

You can even row without a bar.

Press through the center of your feet.

Squeeze your shoulder blades together.

1. Elbow Bridge

Place only the backs of your arms on the floor with your elbows close to the sides of your body. Now push through your elbows and try to lift your upper back and shoulders off the ground and hold that position isometrically for time. You can also do reps up and down, if you'd like. You can make this move easier by fully extending your hips like you would with a Hip Thrust. You can make it harder by fully extending your legs straight in front of your body.

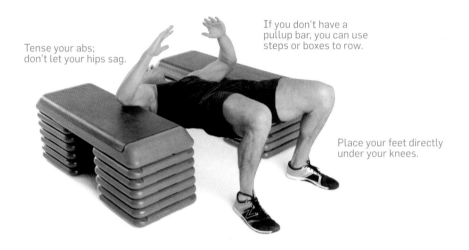

Tense your abs; don't let your hips sag.

If you don't have a pullup bar, you can use steps or boxes to row.

Place your feet directly under your knees.

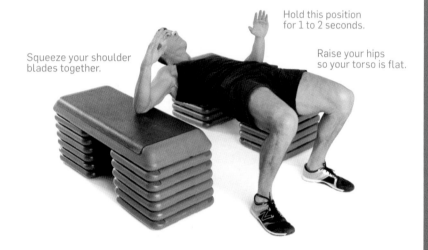

Squeeze your shoulder blades together.

Hold this position for 1 to 2 seconds.

Raise your hips so your torso is flat.

2. Handless Row

Place your body between two chairs, benches, or boxes of even height. Then place your elbows on top of the elevated surfaces. Feel free to place a padded mat, towel, or pillow on the surface to make it more comfortable for your elbows. Next, bend your legs and place your feet directly underneath your knees and then raise your hips until they are fully extended without moving your lower back. Hold this position throughout the movement. Finally, drive your elbows downward as you pull your shoulders down and back and lift your chest up. Once you've gone as far as you can go without letting your shoulders shrug or glide forward, squeeze your shoulder blades together and hold that position for 1 or 2 seconds and then reverse the movement and repeat.

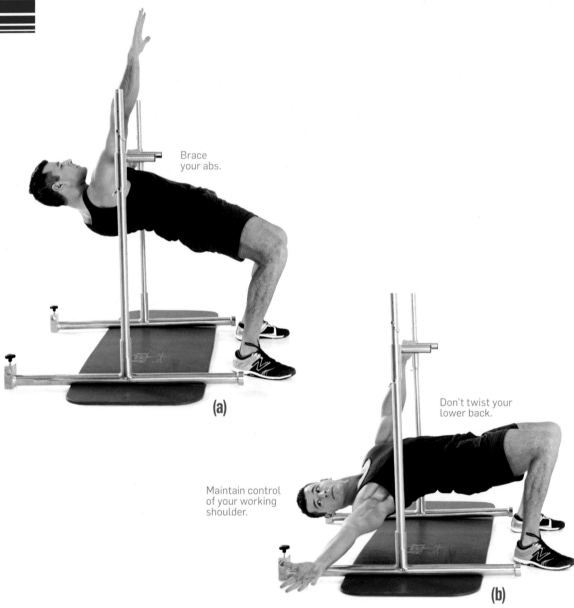

Brace
your abs.

(a)

Don't twist your
lower back.

Maintain control
of your working
shoulder.

(b)

3. Rotating Single-Arm Row

Perform a Single-Arm Row as normal (a), reaching
the nonworking arm toward the ceiling as you pull
up. But as you lower back down, rotate your
upper back (not your lower back) and reach your
nonworking arm down and away from your body (b).

It's critical that you keep the shoulder of your
working arm packed into the socket. You also must
be sure that your hips and shoulders move together
so that you don't twist your lower back.

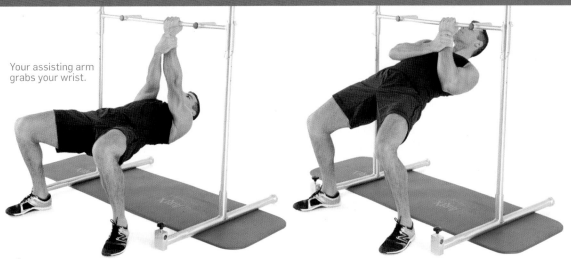

Your assisting arm grabs your wrist.

4. Climber Row

Inspired by the crazy gripping work of rock climbers, this is the most advanced Self-Assisted Single-Arm Row option because one hand is supporting your entire body. Grab the bar or handle with your working arm. Then take your assisting arm and grab the wrist of your working arm. Pull your body up using only as much assistance as you need. Make it harder by moving the assisting hand down toward your elbow, then to your bicep, and eventually to your shoulder.

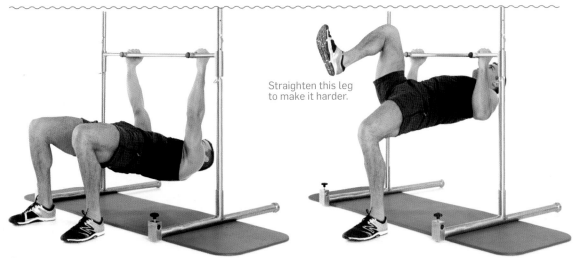

Straighten this leg to make it harder.

5. Spider Row

Another way to shift more work to one side of your body during Rows is to add leg movement. A Spider Row has you flex your hip and bring one knee to the same-side elbow as you pull your body up. Make it even harder by fully extending that same leg to the side at the top position. This shifts more weight to the opposite arm for counterbalance. Perform all of your reps on one side before switching or switch sides every rep.

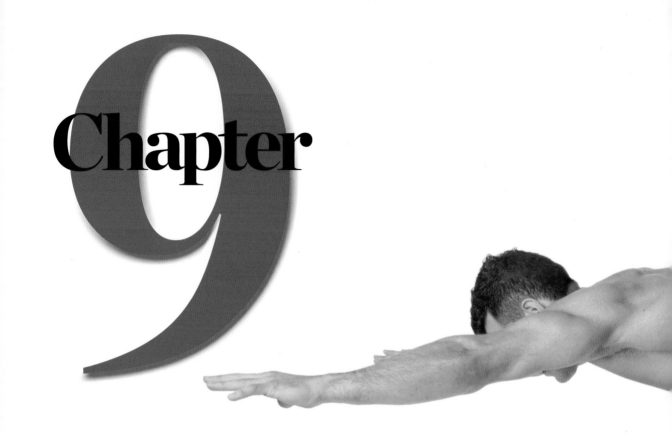

Chapter 9

BODYWEIGHT 8: HIP HINGE

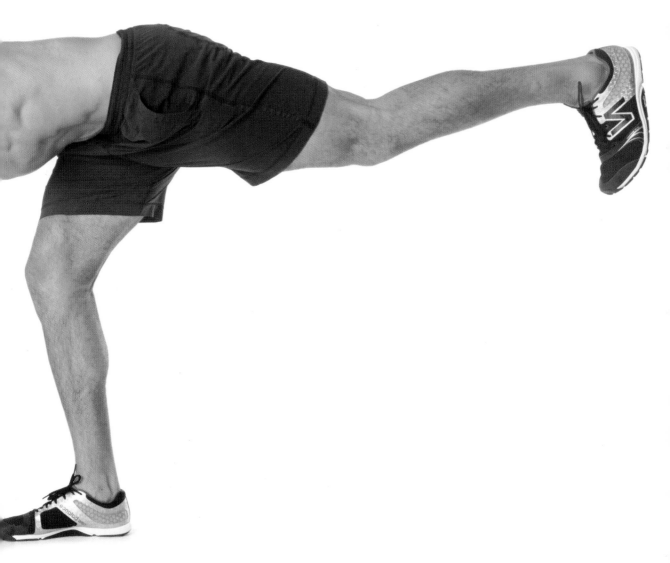

#5 HIP HINGE

The Hip Hinge is the most important bodyweight exercise to master because it works the hips and back side, crucial body parts that are weak and undertrained in most people. Perfecting the technique will help you make every lower-body exercise more hip dominant, and when you do that, you perform it with better form, calling more muscles into play. You'll be able to use your knees through a fuller range of motion. Hip hinging is the stepping-stone to the best fat-burning bodyweight cardio exercises, like Vertical Jumps and Burpees. The progressions in this chapter will provide you with exceptional single-leg balance, lower-back strength, core stability, and hamstring flexibility.

Proper squatting starts by hinging back at your hips. This preloads your hips and hamstrings, allowing you to better keep your knees out, shins vertical, and feet forward—three things critical to the long-term health of your knees. Plus, your hips and hamstrings are stronger than your quads, so if you learn how to recruit them every time you squat (and lunge, step up, or jump), your performance will skyrocket. The key to flawless hip hinging is little to no movement at the knee and lower back. Move only at the hips, keeping a neutral spine. If you suffer from chronic knee issues, Hip Hinges will be your savior. As you try these progressions, remember this one tip, which will make all the difference in understanding what it means to hinge back at your hips: Imagine you are trying to close a door with your butt.

The HIP HINGE Progression

Level 1	Level 2	Level 3	Level 4	Level 5
Ground Zero	Beginner	Intermediate	Advanced	Superhero
HIP HINGE	STAGGERED HIP HINGE	SINGLE-LEG HIP HINGE	VERTICAL JUMP	STAGGERED VERTICAL JUMP

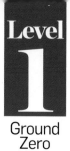

Level 1

Ground Zero

HIP HINGE

Master the Hip Hinge with a parallel foot stance before progressing to more advanced single-leg options. Remember to keep the motion solely at the hips, and do not move your knees or lower back. Only go down as far as you can without moving your lower back, and don't go any lower than the point where your trunk is parallel to the floor. Start with a slight bend in your knees so they are soft. They should not be locked out and fully extended.

ARM POSITION: As you hinge your hips back and bend forward, you can either reach your hands to the floor or extend your hands in front of your body. Even better, place the back of your hands on your lower back; this will stretch your chest and front shoulders and help ensure you maintain a slightly arched lower back.

How to Do It

Starting Position

● Stand with your feet hip- to shoulder-width apart.

● Set your head in a neutral position with your ears aligned with your shoulders, hips, and ankles, and maintain this position as you hinge back and bend forward.

● Assume a hollow-body position: Tense your thighs, glutes, and abs, and push your ribs and shoulders down.

Perfect Execution

● Keep your knees soft with a slight bend, and maintain this position throughout.

● Push your hips and hamstrings back as far as you can (as if closing a door with your butt) until your trunk is parallel to the floor with a slight natural arch in your lower back. You should feel a stretch in the backs of your thighs.

● Briefly pause in the bottom position while maintaining tension throughout your body, then push your hips forward and come to a full stand, being sure to squeeze your glutes at the top of the movement.

Your Goal

You should be able to do multiple sets of 10 reps before moving on to the next level.

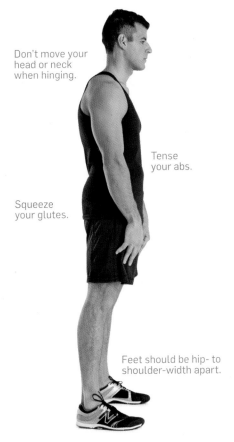

Don't move your head or neck when hinging.

Tense your abs.

Squeeze your glutes.

Feet should be hip- to shoulder-width apart.

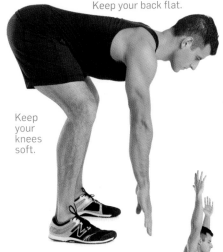

Push your hips back.

Keep your back flat.

Keep your knees soft.

Regressions

MAKE IT EASIER: Hold the bottom position isometrically for time.

EVEN EASIER: Minimize the range of motion as much as needed to maintain a neutral spine position with a slight natural arch in your lower back.

EASIEST: Perform Self-Assisted Hip Hinges by placing your hands on a stable surface that's just below waist height (like a box or bench) that will allow you to get your torso parallel to the floor in the bottom position. Use your hands to help you come up and down.

Progressions

MAKE IT HARDER: Reduce your base of support and increase the range of motion by progressively bringing your feet closer together until they are touching.

EVEN HARDER: Cross your arms with your hands resting on your shoulders (or hold your arms at chest level with your hands in prayer position). From there, place your hands behind your head (prisoner position). Next, fully extend both arms overhead (a).

HARDEST: Combine both of the previous progressions so your feet are together and your arms are overhead for the ultimate test of lower-back strength, core stability, and hamstring flexibility.

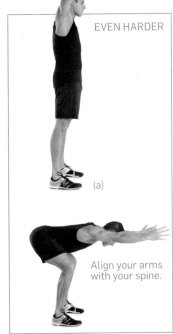

EVEN HARDER

(a)

Align your arms with your spine.

STAGGERED HIP HINGE

Now we're going to stagger your stance to start shifting more weight onto one leg at a time. This will serve as a useful stepping-stone exercise to teach your body what it feels like to keep your hips and shoulders squarely ahead throughout the movement while one leg is doing most of the work. A staggered stance has a leading leg and a trailing leg. The foot of the leading leg is flat on the floor in tripod foot position (as described in Chapter 4). Most of your weight should be on the leading leg. The toes of your trailing leg should be aligned with the heel of your leading leg. Keep your feet about hip-width apart.

How to Do It

Starting Position

• Establish tripod foot position with your leading leg for a natural foot arch with the knuckles of your big toe and little toe and your heel in contact with the ground.

• With your feet hip-width apart, place the toes of your trailing leg on the floor so they are aligned with the heel of your leading leg.

• Keep most of your weight on the leading leg and treat the toes of the trailing leg like the kickstand of a bike.

Perfect Execution

• Keep your knees soft with a slight bend.

• Push your hips and hamstrings back as far as you can (as if closing a door with your butt) until your trunk is parallel to the floor with a slight natural arch in your lower back. You should feel a stretch in the back of the thigh of your leading leg.

• Briefly pause in the bottom position, then push your hips forward and come to a full stand, being sure to squeeze your glutes at the top of the movement.

Your Goal

You should be able to do multiple sets of 10 reps per side before moving on to the next progression.

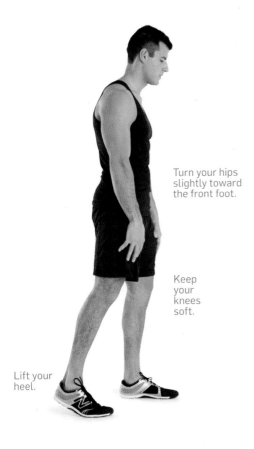

Turn your hips slightly toward the front foot.

Keep your knees soft.

Lift your heel.

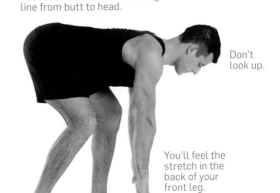

Your back should form a straight line from butt to head.

Don't look up.

You'll feel the stretch in the back of your front leg.

Regressions

MAKE IT EASIER: Hold the bottom position isometrically for time.

EVEN EASIER: Minimize the range of motion as much as needed to maintain a neutral spine position with a slight natural arch in your lower back.

EASIEST: Perform Self-Assisted Staggered Hip Hinges by placing your hands on a stable surface that's just below waist height (like a box or bench) that will allow you to get your torso parallel to the floor in the bottom position. Use your hands to help you come up and down.

Progressions

MAKE IT HARDER: Perform Split Hip Hinges by moving from a staggered stance to a split stance with your trailing leg extended straight behind your body well past your hips.

EVEN HARDER: Perform Rear-Foot-Elevated Staggered Hip Hinges. Elevate your trailing leg on a stable box, bench, bed, or chair of medium height (at or just below knee level). You can also elevate the trailing leg by securing it into the foot cradle of a suspension trainer. This move is unmatched for opening up the hip flexor muscles of your trailing leg.

HARDEST: Do an overhead arms progression by first crossing your arms with your hands resting on your shoulders. From there, place your hands behind your head (prisoner position). Next, fully extend both arms overhead.

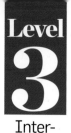

Level

3

Inter-mediate

SINGLE-LEG HIP HINGE

This progression improves your single-leg balance, one of the most neglected fitness qualities to train. No other exercise teaches you how to make your foot one with the ground to properly transfer and absorb ground contact forces all the way up the kinetic chain. The key rule during this movement is to make sure your hips do not rotate away from your working leg. You'll know this has occurred if the toes of your nonworking leg point out to the side as you hinge back at your hips and lower into the bottom position. You can prevent this by squeezing the glute of your nonworking leg throughout the exercise. This will correct your movement by locking your hips into place and corkscrewing your body toward your working leg. It also helps you focus on reaching the heel of your back leg as far away from your body as you can. Be patient with this exercise, because it tends to make newbies really frustrated as they fight for balance.

How to Do It

Starting Position

- Establish tripod foot position with your front foot.
- Screw the foot of your working leg into the floor.
- Turn your hips slightly inward toward your working leg to avoid hip rotation.
- Squeeze the glute of your trailing leg throughout to keep your hips square.

Perfect Execution

- Keep your front knee soft with a slight bend.
- Then push your hips and hamstring back as far as you can (as if closing a door with your butt) until your trunk is parallel to the floor with a slight natural arch in your lower back. You should feel a stretch in the back of the thigh of your leading leg.
- Briefly pause in the bottom position while maintaining tension throughout your body, then push your hips forward and come to a full stand, being sure to squeeze your glutes at the top of the movement.

Your Goal

You should be able to do multiple sets of 10 reps per side before moving on to the next progression.

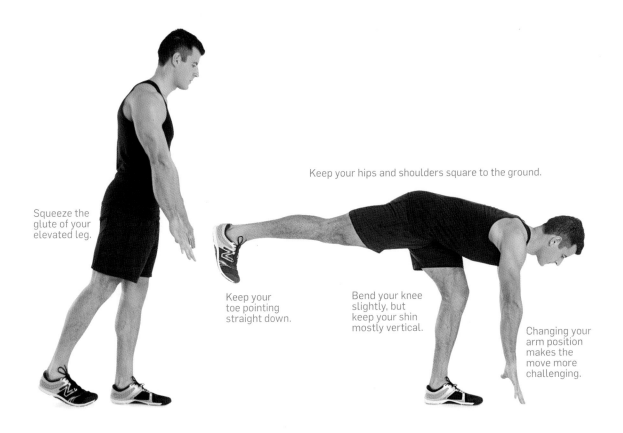

Squeeze the glute of your elevated leg.

Keep your hips and shoulders square to the ground.

Keep your toe pointing straight down.

Bend your knee slightly, but keep your shin mostly vertical.

Changing your arm position makes the move more challenging.

Regressions

MAKE IT EASIER: Simply hold the bottom position isometrically for time.

EVEN EASIER: Minimize the range of motion as much as needed to maintain a neutral spine position with a slight natural arch in your lower back.

EASIEST: Perform Self-Assisted Single-Leg Hip Hinges by placing your hands on a stable surface that's just below waist height (like a table or bench) that will allow you to get your torso parallel to the floor in the bottom position. You can also place one hand against the wall with your side facing the wall, if you'd like. Use your hand(s) to help you come up and down.

Progressions

MAKE IT HARDER: Cross your arms with your hands resting on your shoulders (or hold your arms at chest level with your hands in prayer position).

EVEN HARDER: Perform a Prisoner Single-Leg Hip Hinge by placing your hands behind your head (prisoner position).

HARDEST: Next, perform an Overhead Single-Leg Hip Hinge by fully extending your arms overhead.

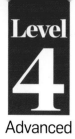
VERTICAL JUMP

Jumping up and down is an unmatched calorie burner. It works every muscle from head to toe and shoots your heart rate through the stratosphere. Jumping for an hour straight is going to cause some serious fat loss and really tax your cardiovascular system, but at what expense? Jumping improperly will wear down your joints quickly. The solution? Learning how to land properly with your knees out, shins vertical, and toes pointing straight ahead. Most people don't get injured from jumping, they get injured from lousy landings.

Vertical jumping is driven through your posterior chain—the muscles of your spine, hips, hamstrings, and calves. To engage these powerful muscles, you must stretch and load your hips like you do with a Hip Hinge. In fact, vertical jumping is basically explosive hip hinging. Though most of the movement is driven through your hips, it's okay to bend your knees slightly when jumping up and landing. Just don't bend your knees too much; otherwise, it becomes more of a Jump Squat (see Chapter 7). The more you move your hips and the less you move your knees, the easier it will be on your knees.

How to Do It

Starting Position

- Establish tripod foot position with both feet.

- Set your head in a neutral position with your ears aligned with your shoulders, hips, and ankles as you hinge back and bend.

- Extend your arms overhead, tense your thighs, glutes, and abs, and push your ribs and shoulders down.

Perfect Execution

- Load for a jump by hinging back at your hips, bending your trunk forward, and extending your arms behind your body.

- Briefly pause in the bottom position. Then push your hips forward to fully extend your knees, swing your arms overhead, and push away from the ground with your toes to extend your ankles.

- Land softly into the loaded hinged-squat position on the balls of your feet and get your knees out, shins vertical, and feet forward.

- Take your time to reset to the starting position. Hold the landings for a couple seconds before performing continuous repetitions.

Your Goal

You should be able to do multiple sets of 10 reps with soft landings.

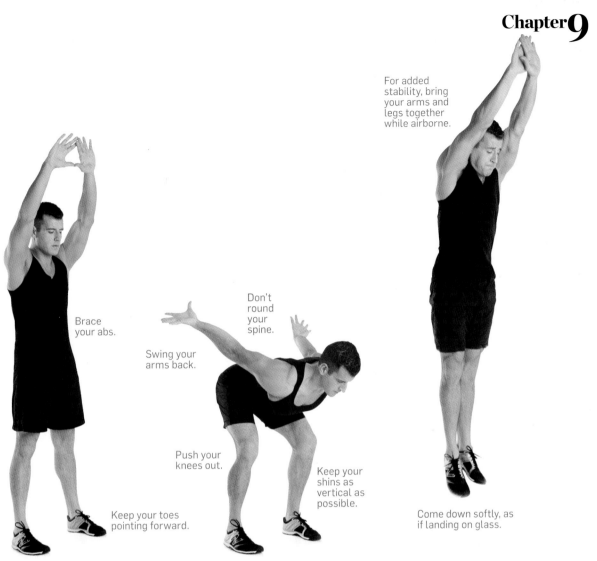

For added stability, bring your arms and legs together while airborne.

Brace your abs.

Don't round your spine.

Swing your arms back.

Push your knees out.

Keep your shins as vertical as possible.

Keep your toes pointing forward.

Come down softly, as if landing on glass.

Regressions

MAKE IT EASIER: Don't jump up as high. and perform the movement more slowly.

EVEN EASIER: Only jump up high enough that a piece of paper could slide underneath your feet.

EASIEST: Perform explosive calf raises where you simply come up on your toes as high as you can without letting your feet leave the floor. This is the best way for beginners to start learning good jumping and landing mechanics. They are very useful for higher reps and short rest periods, even for advanced trainees.

Progressions

MAKE IT HARDER: Accelerate the jumping phase by really ripping your arms upward.

EVEN HARDER: Next, accelerate the loading phase by really ripping your arms down and back to increase the stretched-rubber-band effect of your muscles and connective tissues for more explosive jumping.

HARDEST: Once you can stick and hold the landings with perfect form, progress to continuous jumps where you immediately jump back up as soon as you land into the hinged-squat position. This increases the metabolic demands of the exercise. This variation is meant for advanced trainees and develops greater elasticity.

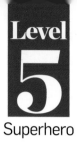

STAGGERED VERTICAL JUMP

This is just like a Vertical Jump on two legs except we increase the challenge by progressively shifting more of the work toward one leg at a time. You'll start with a staggered stance to bridge the gap between jumping on two legs and jumping on one leg. Then you'll use microprogressions to gradually build up to the real deal: Single-Leg Vertical Jumps. This is the king of explosive total-body bodyweight exercises and will make you a freakish athlete (in a good way, of course). If you can jump and land flawlessly on one leg, you can do just about anything with your lower body. Oh yeah, get good at these and you'll be jumping through the rafters on both legs. If you want to be able to dunk a basketball and you're not exceptionally tall, this move is a must.

How to Do It

Starting Position

- Establish tripod position with your leading foot.

- With your feet hip-width apart, place the toes of your trailing leg on the floor so they are aligned with the heel of your leading leg.

- Keep most of your weight on the leading leg.

Perfect Execution

- Load up for a jump by hinging back at your hips, bending forward, and extending your arms behind your body.

- Briefly pause in the bottom position, then push your hips forward to fully extend your hips and knees, swing your arms overhead, and push away from the ground with your toes to fully extend your ankles.

- Land softly into the loaded hinged-squat position in that same staggered stance on the balls of your feet.

- Take your time to reset to the starting position, almost treating each rep as a separate set. Focus on holding the landings for a couple seconds before performing continuous repetitions.

Your Goal

You should be able to do multiple sets of 10 reps per side with soft landings.

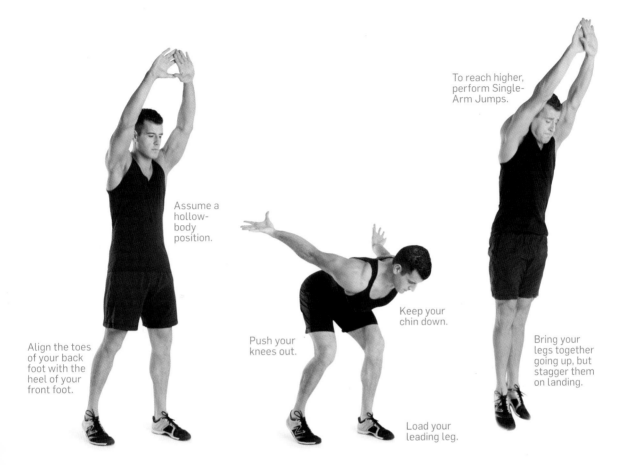

To reach higher, perform Single-Arm Jumps.

Assume a hollow-body position.

Keep your chin down.

Align the toes of your back foot with the heel of your front foot.

Push your knees out.

Load your leading leg.

Bring your legs together going up, but stagger them on landing.

Regressions

MAKE IT EASIER: Don't jump up as high and perform the movement more slowly.

EVEN EASIER: Only jump up high enough that a piece of paper could slide underneath your feet.

EASIEST: Perform explosive calf raises where you simply come up on your toes as high as you can without letting your feet leave the floor. This is the best way for beginners to start learning good jumping and landing mechanics. They are very useful for higher reps and short rest periods, even for advanced trainees.

Progressions

MAKE IT HARDER: Jump up on one leg and land on two legs to start prepping your body for Single-Leg Vertical Jumps. Start with slower and smaller jumps and build to faster and bigger jumps.

EVEN HARDER: Perform Single-Leg Vertical Jumps by jumping and landing on one leg. Be sure to hold the landing for a couple seconds before resetting for the next rep. Treat each rep as if it's a separate set.

HARDEST: Progress to continuous Single-Leg Jumps where you immediately jump back up as soon as you land into the hinged-squat position. This increases the metabolic demands of the exercise, and is meant for advanced trainees to develop greater elasticity.

Variations

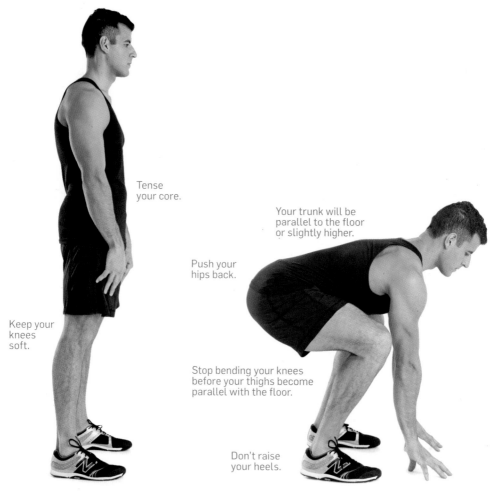

Tense
your core.

Your trunk will be
parallel to the floor
or slightly higher.

Push your
hips back.

Keep your
knees
soft.

Stop bending your knees
before your thighs become
parallel with the floor.

Don't raise
your heels.

1. Hinging Squat

Stand with your feet hip- to shoulder-width apart
and assume a hollow-body posture. As you push
your hips back (as if closing a door with your butt),
bend your knees. You can touch the floor with your
fingertips and then progress further by touching
the floor with your palms to increase the range of
motion. This is an excellent exercise modification
for those with painful knees because it still works
the squatting pattern while putting almost all of
the work on the hips and hamstrings. It will also
work the quads, without involving deep knee bends.

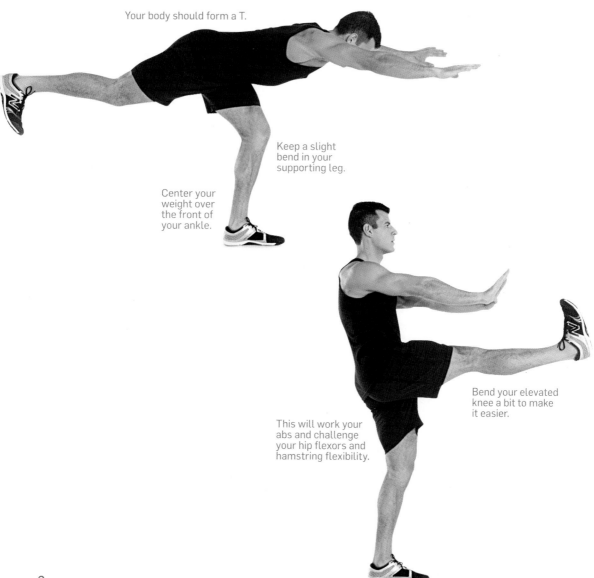

Your body should form a T.

Keep a slight bend in your supporting leg.

Center your weight over the front of your ankle.

Bend your elevated knee a bit to make it easier.

This will work your abs and challenge your hip flexors and hamstring flexibility.

2. Single-Leg Hip Hinge and Leg Raise

This is the ultimate test of single-leg balance, and it works every muscle on the front, back, inside, and outside of your hips. Stand straight with feet shoulder-width apart in hollow-body position, your arms extended in front of you. As you hinge back at the hips, simultaneously bend forward and raise your right leg straight behind you. Balance in that position for 2 seconds, then raise your torso back up while raising your right leg in front of you. Do all reps and then switch legs or alternate each rep with a different leg. Be sure to avoid rounding your back throughout the exercise.

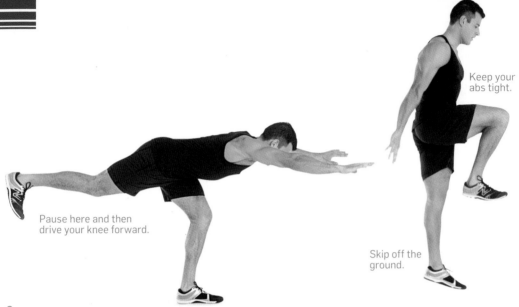

Pause here and then drive your knee forward.

Keep your abs tight.

Skip off the ground.

3. Single-Leg Hip Hinge and Jump

Perform a Single-Leg Hip Hinge as usual but as you return to the standing position, explode through your hips and drive the knee of your nonsupporting leg upward as you go slightly airborne as if skipping. Land softly, and repeat. After completing your reps, switch to the other leg.

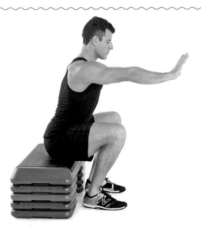
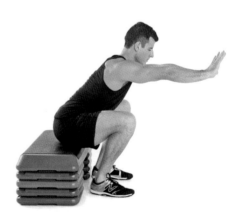

4. Seated Hip Hinge

This mobility variation allows you to isolate the hip-hinging movement without the balance demands that come with being on your feet. Start by sitting tall in a chair or on a box with your abs braced and your ribs and shoulders down. Then hinge forward at your hips until your belly and ribs press into your thighs without allowing your lower back to round. Finish by pushing your hips forward until you're back in a tall seated position. You can choose among various chair or box heights.

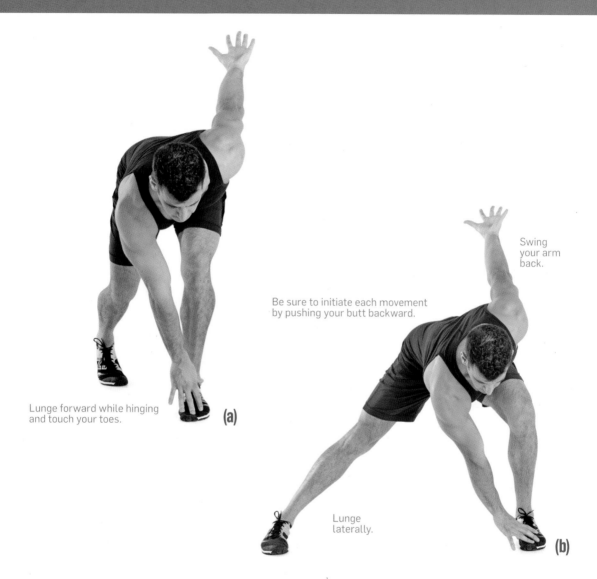

Be sure to initiate each movement by pushing your butt backward.

Swing your arm back.

Lunge forward while hinging and touch your toes. (a)

Lunge laterally. (b)

5. Hinging Lunge

This is the same concept as the Hinging Squat (variation 1). You're going to hinge at your hips until your trunk is parallel to the floor or slightly higher and also bend a bit at the knee. The Lunge step tends to be smaller and more contained within your center of gravity. You can step forward (a), backward, or to the side (b); cross over or under; or even take a rotational step. All of these variations serve to make your hips and hamstrings work harder and take pressure off of your knees while still allowing for some knee movement and a little more quad work. These types of Lunges tend to be more applicable to daily activities and sports because you need to bend over more often than you need to sink into Deep Squat positions. It's also a more efficient stepping pattern.

BODYWEIGHT 8: HANDSTAND PUSHUP

Chapter 10

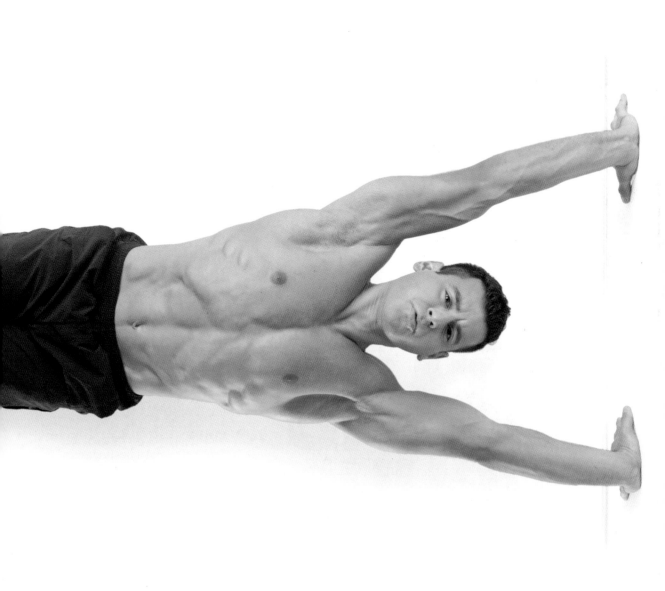

#6
HAND-STAND PUSHUP

If you're looking for the best way to sculpt the shoulders of a superhero, this wins hands down.

The vertical pressing pattern of the Handstand Pushup forces you to support 100 percent of your body weight as opposed to only 70 percent with traditional floor Pushups. Sound tough? Thinking there's no way you'll be able to do these moves? Well, that's where step-by-step exercise progression comes into play.

It's all about adjusting your body angle as much as needed so you can safely train the muscles that push your arms overhead. And here's a nice incentive for doing the work: Making your shoulders wider and more developed will automatically make you look leaner by causing your waist to appear smaller from every angle.

Caution: Supporting your body weight with your hands over your head requires a great deal of shoulder mobility and core stability. People who struggle to get their arms overhead will often compensate by arching and extending their lower back and shrugging and elevating their shoulders. This is a recipe for shoulder and back pain. Will you have that trouble? Test yourself right now by putting your back against a wall with your head, upper back, and butt making contact and your arms at your sides. Your feet should be as close to the wall as your butt allows. Assume a hollow-body position and then slowly raise your straight arms in front of you and overhead while keeping your ribs and shoulders down and core braced. Stop raising your arms the moment you start to lose the hollow-body position and begin to hyperextend your lower back. If you can't touch the wall with your hands, it means you're missing flexion motion at the shoulder and not ready for the advanced exercises in this chapter. I encourage everyone to use the step-by-step progressions to gain the mandatory mobility.

There are ample benefits to Handstand Pushups besides making you as strong on your hands as most people are on their feet (pretty cool, right?). Hand balancing (or arm balancing, as some call it) strengthens your hands, mobilizes your wrists, and improves your overall sense of balance and body awareness. Inversion (being upside down) improves your digestion and circulation and brings more blood to your brain. Kicking up into a Handstand against a wall and holding the top position for as long as you can is a great daily habit to maximize your overall health and performance. Just be sure to take your shoes off so you don't mark the wall!

The HANDSTAND PUSHUP Progression

Level 1	Level 2	Level 3	Level 4	Level 5
Ground Zero	Beginner	Intermediate	Advanced	Superhero
DIRTY DOG PUSHUP	PUSH-AWAY	PIKE PUSHUP	HANDSTAND PUSHUP	SELF-ASSISTED SINGLE-ARM HANDSTAND PUSHUP

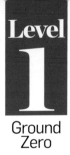

DIRTY DOG PUSHUP

Probably the most basic and popular pose in yoga is the Downward Dog, where you begin in a Pushup position and then push your hips back as far as you can. It's a natural stretch that four-legged animals do every day. My two boxers, Mustafa and Kaila, hit this mobility move every time they wake up or stand from a lying position, which seems to be a hundred times a day. (Hint to humans!) There is no better way to open your shoulders and hips in one fell swoop and instantly feel better. This move simultaneously stretches the entire back side of your body while activating the front. It lengthens your calves and hamstrings (which takes pressure off your back and knees) and it opens up your shoulder girdle (which improves posture).

But there's more to this basic stretch. It's a great warmup move for workouts or sports and an anytime, anywhere full-body energizer when you're feeling flat. Quick note: Unlike yoga's Downward Dog, the Dirty Dog should be performed with feet together, if possible, as this will best translate to the other progressions. However, if you have poor hamstring flexibility, you may need to widen your feet or even bend your knees slightly to fully execute this movement.

How to Do It

Starting Position

- Place your hands directly underneath your shoulders with arms extended.

- Screw your hands into the floor and grip the ground with your fingertips.

- Set your head in a neutral position with your ears aligned with your shoulders, hips, and ankles, and gaze between your hands.

- Assume a hollow-body Pushup position with your feet together: Squeeze your legs together, tense your thighs, glutes, and abs, and pull your ribs and shoulders down.

Perfect Execution

- Hinge at your hips and push your butt back as far as you can while keeping your arms fully extended and trying to get your feet flat on the floor.

- Briefly hold this position and sink into the stretch. Push your head as far away from your hands as possible while keeping your chest up. Reverse the movement and then perform a full-range-of-motion Pushup if you can and repeat.

Your Goal

You should be able to do multiple sets of 10 reps before moving to the next level.

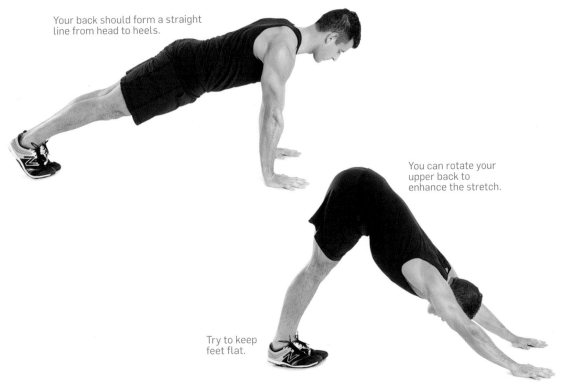

Your back should form a straight line from head to heels.

You can rotate your upper back to enhance the stretch.

Try to keep feet flat.

Regressions

MAKE IT EASIER: If you're not strong enough to do a floor Pushup while in the top position, skip it and just hold the Plank position briefly before shifting back into the stretching portion.

EVEN EASIER: Increase your base of support by widening your hands or feet.

EASIEST: Decrease your body angle by performing a Hands-Elevated Dirty Dog. Place your hands on a sturdy box, bench, chair, or ottoman. It's best to place this object against a wall so that it doesn't slide on you when pushing back. This makes it much easier because you're holding less of your body weight.

Progressions

MAKE IT HARDER: Progressively bring your hands closer together until your thumbs are touching.

EVEN HARDER: Perform Single-Leg Dirty Dogs (a). Lift one leg off of the floor and squeeze the glute of your supporting leg while driving the toes into the floor.

HARDEST: Perform Single-Arm Dirty Dogs (b). Place the hand of your working arm directly underneath your shoulder or slightly inward toward your body's midline before hinging back. Move your other hand to your back. Place your feet shoulder-width apart or wider for balance.

SUPER HARD: Raise the leg opposite your nonworking arm (c).

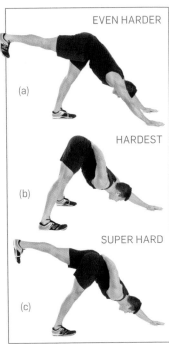

EVEN HARDER

(a)

HARDEST

(b)

SUPER HARD

(c)

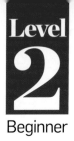
PUSH-AWAY

This stepping-stone exercise works the angle in between horizontal and vertical pushing while putting a greater load through your shoulders than Dirty Dogs do. It's a perfect mix between a regular Pushup and the Pike Pushup to be shown in Level 3. If you're doing it right, you should feel it mostly in your shoulders and less in your chest. Focus on keeping your hips higher than your shoulders throughout the movement.

How to Do It

Starting Position

- Get into the Dirty Dog position with your hips piked up and pushed back toward your feet and your arms fully extended in front of you.

- Screw your hands into the floor and grip the ground with your fingertips.

- Spread your fingers as wide as you can with your fingertips pointing straight ahead.

- Set your head in a neutral position with your ears aligned with your shoulders, hips, and ankles, and keep your gaze centered between your hands.

Perfect Execution

- Bend your elbows and shift your body as far forward as you can until your head passes through your hands and your nose touches the floor.

- Briefly pause in this position, feeling your shoulders work, and then push back and away (not straight up), reversing the movement to return to the starting position.

- Keep your hips higher than your shoulders throughout the movement.

Your Goal

You should be able to do multiple sets of 10 reps before moving to the next level.

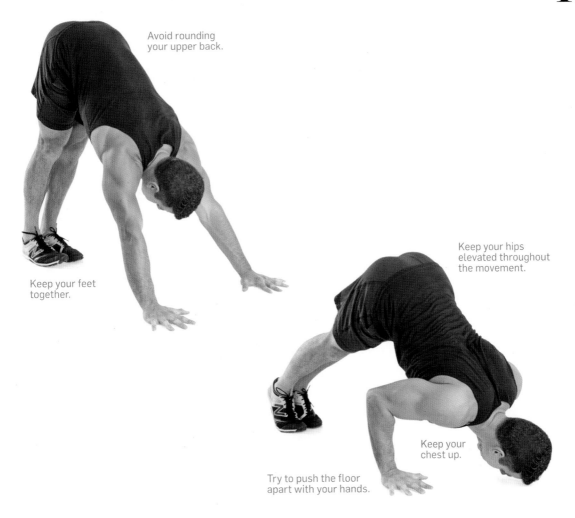

Avoid rounding your upper back.

Keep your feet together.

Keep your hips elevated throughout the movement.

Keep your chest up.

Try to push the floor apart with your hands.

Regressions

MAKE IT EASIER: Increase your base of support by widening your feet.

EVEN EASIER: Increase your base of support and decrease the range of motion by widening your hands.

EASIEST: Decrease your body angle by performing the Hands-Elevated Push-Away. Place your hands on a sturdy box, bench, chair, ottoman, or even a wall. This makes it much easier because you're holding less of your body weight.

Progressions

MAKE IT HARDER: Perform the Close-Grip Push-Away. Progressively bring your hands closer together until your thumbs touch.

EVEN HARDER: Perform Single-Leg Push-Aways. Lift one leg off of the floor and squeeze the glute of your supporting leg while driving the toes into the floor to keep your hips square to the ground.

HARDEST: Perform the Single-Arm Push-Away. Place the hand of your working arm directly underneath your same-side shoulder or slightly inward toward your body's midline. Place your feet shoulder-width apart or wider for extra balance.

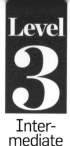

PIKE PUSHUP

This is your first foray into the inverted Pushups, in which your upper body is upside down. If you do a Pike Pushup with your feet on the floor, the easier option, only your upper body will be inverted. If you do it with your feet elevated on a stable surface that's at about hip level, then your whole body will be inverted. The feet-elevated option is almost as challenging to your shoulders as Handstand Pushups, except that your hands aren't supporting as much of your leg mass. It's also a lot easier on your abs (and lower back) because your knees are bent and behind your body, and it doesn't require as much balance as when your legs are fully extended overhead. Feel free to place a padded mat or pillow underneath your body so that you can have a soft target for your head in the beginning.

How to Do It

Starting Position

- Place your feet together and on a stable box, bench, chair, step, or ottoman at shin to hip height. Your hips should be aligned over your hands, head, and shoulders.

- Keep your weight over the center of your hands (just in front of your wrists).

- Screw your hands into the floor and grip the ground with your fingertips.

- Spread your fingers as wide as you can with your fingertips pointing straight ahead.

- Set your head in a neutral position with your ears aligned with your shoulders, hips, and ankles.

Perfect Execution

- Bend your elbows and slowly lower your head to the floor. Don't bounce your head off the floor!

- Briefly pause in this position, feeling your shoulders work, and then push up and away to reverse the movement and return to the starting position.

- Keep your pelvis balanced over your ribs throughout the movement.

Your Goal

You should be able to do multiple sets of 10 reps before moving to the next level.

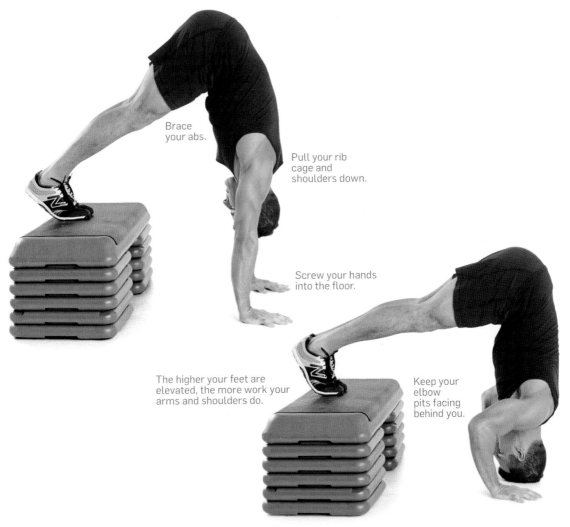

Brace
your abs.

Pull your rib
cage and
shoulders down.

Screw your hands
into the floor.

The higher your feet are
elevated, the more work your
arms and shoulders do.

Keep your
elbow
pits facing
behind you.

Regressions

MAKE IT EASIER: Decrease your body angle and place your feet on the floor so you're pushing and supporting less of your body weight.

EVEN EASIER: Increase your base of support and decrease the range of motion by widening your hands.

EASIEST: Perform a Pike Pushup Hold with your arms fully extended. This will help you build the shoulder strength and core stability needed to perform the actual Pushup component.

Progressions

MAKE IT HARDER: Perform Single-Leg Pike Pushups. Lift one leg off the box or floor and extend that leg upward as much as you can to simulate the leg positioning of a Handstand Pushup.

EVEN HARDER: Increase the range of motion with Close-Grip Pike Pushups. Progressively bring your hands closer together until your thumbs touch.

HARDEST: Increase the range of motion by placing your hands on elevated surfaces of even height like two low steps/boxes, balls, weight plates, or books. This will allow your head to sink lower than the floor would otherwise allow.

HANDSTAND PUSHUP

Warning: Don't attempt this difficult move until you've mastered the previous progressions.

This is the ultimate shoulder builder and a true test of your core because your legs are fully extended overhead, which makes your abs work to prevent your lower back from arching too much. You must first master the ability to kick your legs up to the wall. Do so by placing your hands on the floor 6 to 12 inches in front of a sturdy wall with one foot forward and one foot back. The forward leg should be bent and the back leg should be fully extended. Then kick up into a Handstand one leg at a time by pressing off with your trailing leg. Do your best to come up slowly and with control so that your legs don't smash into the wall like a wrecking ball. Focus on keeping your arms fully locked out and extended throughout the kick up. Where people can get into trouble is if they panic and then let their arms bend, which puts you at risk of falling on your head. Until you become proficient, use a safety spotter to assist you in getting into position and performing the exercise.

Another note of caution: The top of your head should touch, *never bounce,* off the floor. And never hyperextend your neck.

How to Do It

Starting Position

• Place your hands on the floor 6 to 12 inches in front of a sturdy wall and then kick up into a Handstand one leg at a time.

• Keep your weight over the center of your hands (just in front of your wrists).

• Screw your hands into the floor and grip the ground with your fingertips.

• Spread your fingertips as wide as you can.

• Assume a hollow-body position with your feet together and your toes pointing up. Squeeze your legs together, tense your thighs, glutes, and abs, and pull your ribs and shoulders down.

Perfect Execution

• Bend your elbows and slowly lower the top of your head to the floor. Do not let your head hit the floor!

• Briefly pause, feeling your shoulders work, and then push up and away to the starting position.

• Keep your pelvis balanced over your ribs throughout the movement.

• Bring your legs down slowly one at a time when exiting the Handstand.

Your Goal

You should be able to do multiple sets of 10 reps before moving to the next level.

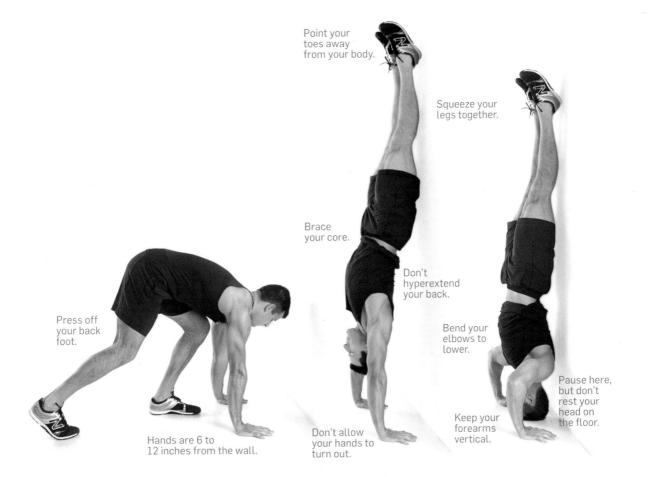

Point your toes away from your body.

Squeeze your legs together.

Brace your core.

Don't hyperextend your back.

Press off your back foot.

Bend your elbows to lower.

Hands are 6 to 12 inches from the wall.

Don't allow your hands to turn out.

Keep your forearms vertical.

Pause here, but don't rest your head on the floor.

Regressions

MAKE IT EASIER: Increase your base of support by widening your feet.

EVEN EASIER: Increase your base of support and decrease the range of motion by widening your hands.

EASIEST: Simply perform a Handstand Hold with your arms fully extended. This will help you build the shoulder strength and core stability needed to perform the actual Pushup component.

Progressions

MAKE IT HARDER: Perform Single-Leg Handstand Pushups with only one foot in contact with the wall. Focus on squeezing your glutes to prevent lower-back hyperextension.

EVEN HARDER: Increase the range of motion by performing Close-Grip Handstand Pushups. Progressively bring your hands closer together until your thumbs are touching.

HARDEST: Increase the range of motion by placing your hands on independently elevated surfaces of even height like two weight plates or books. This will allow your head to sink lower than the floor would otherwise allow.

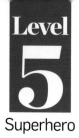
SELF-ASSISTED SINGLE-ARM HANDSTAND PUSHUP

Now it's time to start shifting more of the work to one side of your body at a time. I should probably mention that very few people in the world can pull this move off with full range of motion and perfect form on one arm without some significant off-arm assistance. As of the time of writing this book, I'm not one of them. Still, we need a way to independently train one arm or shoulder at a time like we could with a Single-Arm Dumbbell Shoulder Press. That's why we're going to be using self-assisted versions so that everyone can reap the rewards of unilateral training. Start with Self-Assisted Single-Arm Push-Aways first before progressing to the Pike and Handstand versions.

How to Do It

Starting Position

● Kick up into a two-hand Handstand as described in Level 4. You may want to set up in the corner of a wall so each foot can press off of the edges for extra stability.

● Once you secure the hollow-body position with your feet together, shift your weight to one hand (your working arm) and come up onto the fingertips of your other hand (your assisting arm). This is a staggered-hand setup.

Perfect Execution

● Bend your elbows and slowly lower the top of your head to the floor, keeping most of your weight on your working arm. Do not let your head bounce off the floor!

● Briefly pause in this position, feeling your shoulders work, and then push up and away to return to the starting position. Only use as much assistance from your assisting arm as needed.

● Bring your legs down slowly. It tends to be easier to come down one leg at a time.

Your Goal

You should be able to do multiple sets of 10 reps per side.

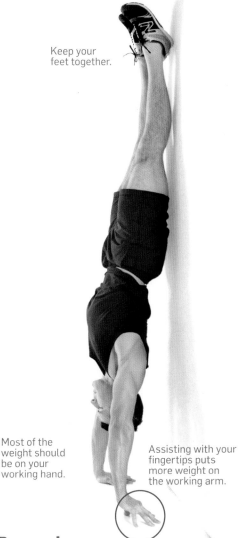

Keep your feet together.

Most of the weight should be on your working hand.

Assisting with your fingertips puts more weight on the working arm.

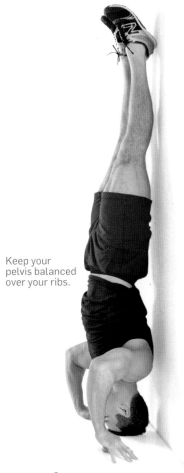

Keep your pelvis balanced over your ribs.

Regressions

MAKE IT EASIER: Perform Self-Assisted Single-Arm Pike Pushups.

EVEN EASIER: Perform Self-Assisted Single-Arm Push-Aways.

EASIEST: Perform Single-Arm Dirty Dogs.

Progressions

MAKE IT HARDER: Perform an Archer Handstand Pushup where the hand of the assisting arm is fully extended to the side of your body, just like with an Archer Pushup.

EVEN HARDER: Perform the Single-Arm Handstand Pushup Hold without assistance. This is best done in the corner of a wall to allow your feet to press off of the edges so that they don't slip to the side as much.

HARDEST: Perform the Single-Arm Handstand Pushup. Progress further by performing this move freestanding without the support and assistance of a wall. If you can pull this off, your body is basically functioning like it's in a zero-gravity environment.

Variations

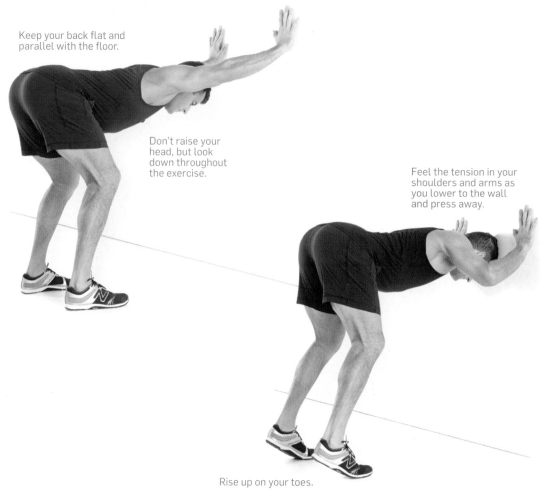

Keep your back flat and parallel with the floor.

Don't raise your head, but look down throughout the exercise.

Feel the tension in your shoulders and arms as you lower to the wall and press away.

Rise up on your toes.

1. Wall Push-Away

An easy way for beginners to mimic the movement of the Handstand Pushup is by pushing the body away from a wall. Stand about 3 feet away from a sturdy wall with feet shoulder-width apart. Hinge your hips back, bend your knees slightly, and bend forward with arms outstretched until your hands contact the wall. Keep your back flat. Now bend your elbows to bring your head to the wall. Rise up on your toes to press into the wall. Pause, then straighten your arms against the resistance of your legs pushing forward. Keep your body hinged, and repeat.

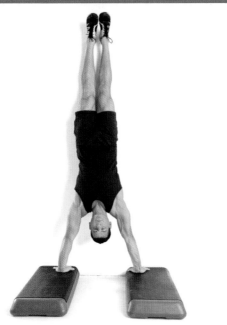

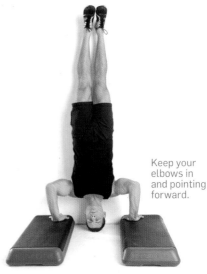

Keep your
elbows in
and pointing
forward.

2. Extended-Range-of-Motion Handstand Pushup

Place your hands on two low boxes, steps, or even phone books of even height to allow your head to lower farther than it would if your hands were on the floor. This increased range of motion creates an extra challenge for your shoulder muscles. Make it easier by doing it from the Pike position with your feet elevated or on the floor.

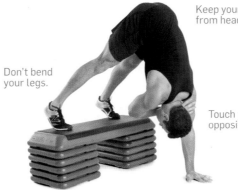

Keep your back flat
from head to tailbone.

Don't bend
your legs.

Touch your
opposite shoulder.

3. Pike Shoulder Tap

Build bolder shoulders by shifting your weight to one hand and then picking up the other hand and touching the opposite shoulder while in the Pike Pushup position. Reverse the movement, switch sides, and repeat. This move is best performed slowly for more stability and control. Add a Pike Pushup between reps if you're up for it. Make it harder by doing it from the Handstand position against a wall.

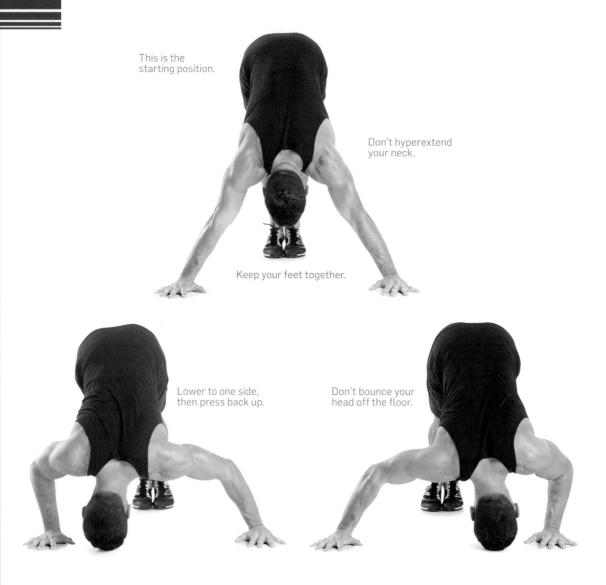

This is the
starting position.

Don't hyperextend
your neck.

Keep your feet together.

Lower to one side,
then press back up.

Don't bounce your
head off the floor.

4. Side-to-Side Pike Pushup

Begin this exercise as a normal Pike Pushup but as you lower your body to the ground, slowly shift your weight as much to one side as you can. Then push back up to the starting position. You can either switch sides every rep or perform all of your reps on one side before switching.

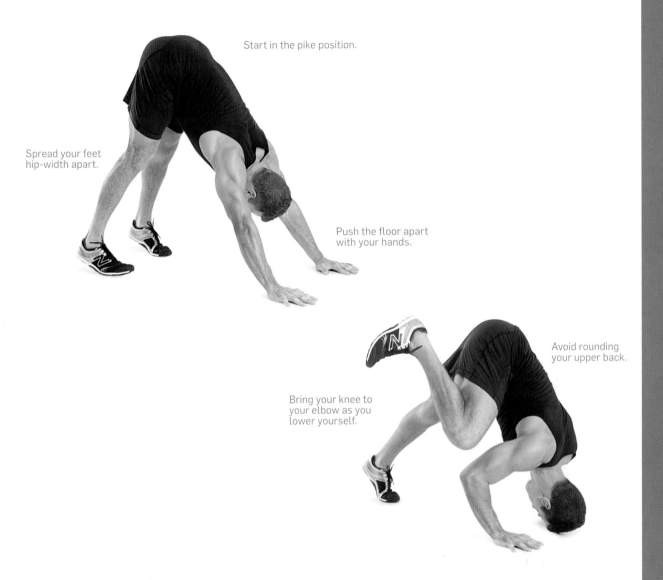

Start in the pike position.

Spread your feet hip-width apart.

Push the floor apart with your hands.

Avoid rounding your upper back.

Bring your knee to your elbow as you lower yourself.

5. Spider Pike Pushup

Another way to shift more work to one side of your body during Pike Pushups is to add leg movement. As with a Spider Pushup, flex your hip and bring one knee to the same-side elbow as you lower to the bottom position. You can make it even harder by fully extending that same leg to the side in the bottom position. This forces you to shift more weight to the opposite arm for counterbalance. You can either perform all of your reps on one side before switching or switch sides every rep.

BODYWEIGHT 8: SINGLE-LEG SQUAT

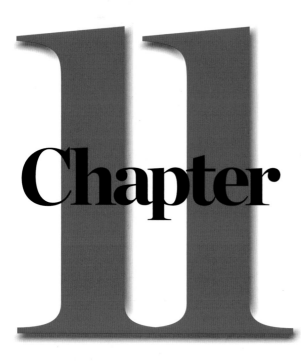

Chapter

11

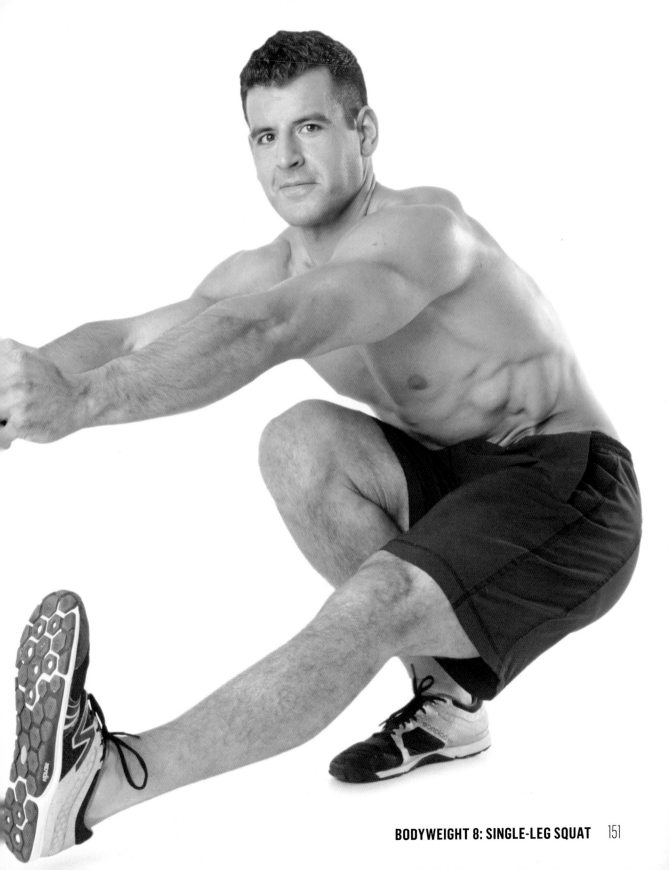

#7
7
SINGLE-LEG SQUAT

There is a huge achievement gap between squatting on both legs and squatting on one leg. The former requires squatting half of your body weight on each leg with a larger base of support and two points of contact. The latter requires squatting all of your body weight on one leg with a smaller base of support and only one point of contact. It's a night-and-day difference for the muscles of your lower body (and your nervous system), and that's why a system of smart exercise progressions to bridge this *ginormous* strength and stability gap is a must.

Single-Leg Squats are so beneficial because they train all of your lower-body muscles in three planes of motion. As your body performs the movement up and down, it must fight lateral and rotational forces. Standing on one leg requires all of the muscles on the inside and outside of your hips and thighs to activate to stabilize your knees and your core muscles to kick in to stabilize your spine. If you really think about it, a Single-Leg Squat is basically a Standing Plank on one leg.

Most of what we do throughout the day or during athletic activities like walking and running takes place one leg at a time. That's why it's critical to practice both Squats on two legs and Squats on one leg.

All of us have strength and flexibility imbalances between sides. If all you do is Squats on two legs, you'll proliferate these imbalances, which leads to dysfunctional movement, and increased risk of injury. The better you get at squatting on one leg, the better you'll get at squatting on two. In general, perform 2 to 3 sets on your weak leg for every set you perform on your strong leg to help quickly correct an imbalance between sides.

The SINGLE-LEG SQUAT Progression

Level 1	Level 2	Level 3	Level 4	Level 5
Ground Zero	Beginner	Intermediate	Advanced	Superhero
SINGLE-LEG WALL SIT	STEPUP	STAGGERED SQUAT	LUNGE	SINGLE-LEG SQUAT

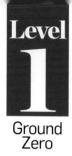
SINGLE-LEG WALL SIT

The Single-Leg Wall Sit is an exercise that anybody can do, especially when modifying the range of motion by raising the hips above knee level as much as needed. It's a safe, stable, and low-skill way to set up in a Single-Leg Squat position with perfect posture. The upright and vertical trunk position shifts a greater emphasis to your quads, helping you build up all of the muscles surrounding your knee to ensure that your patella tracks properly. This is especially important for people with a history of knee pain. Isometric holds are also easier on your joints than dynamic full-range-of-motion repetitions. Though this move is categorized as an entry-level exercise, it can continue to be used by more advanced trainees for warmups, active recovery, or endurance work. Plus, if you sink low enough so that your hips are below knee level, this move will challenge anyone.

How to Do It

Starting Position

- Stand with your back to a wall with your feet about hip-width apart or closer and arms extended. Your heels should be about 2 feet from the wall.

- Establish tripod foot position with your feet together.

- Sit into a Squat position with your hips making a 90-degree angle and your hips, upper back, and head in full contact with the wall.

Perfect Execution

- Slowly shift your weight to the working leg as you pick up your nonworking leg.

- Sit as tall as possible and hold this position for time while keeping your hips and shoulders square for the full duration.

- If you fatigue before time is up, simply decrease the range of motion as much as needed midset to keep going.

- After 60 seconds, repeat on the other leg.

Your Goal

You should be able to hold a Single-Leg Wall Sit for multiple sets of 60 seconds on each leg with your hips below knee level before moving to the next level.

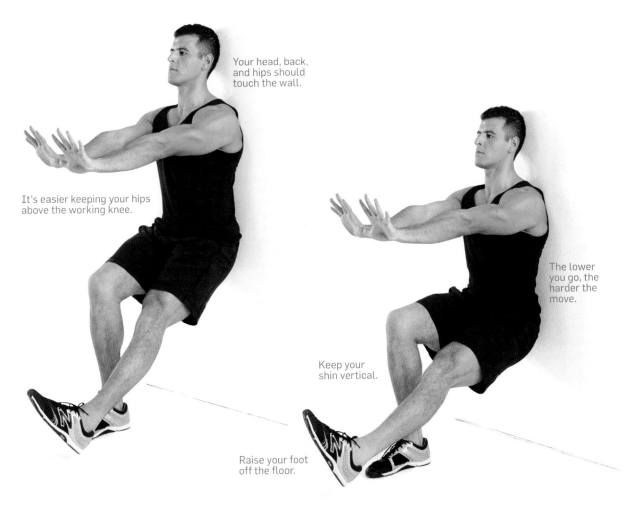

Your head, back, and hips should touch the wall.

It's easier keeping your hips above the working knee.

The lower you go, the harder the move.

Keep your shin vertical.

Raise your foot off the floor.

Regressions

MAKE IT EASIER: Perform an alternating Wall Sit March, switching legs every few seconds.

EVEN EASIER: Decrease the range of motion so that your hips are higher than knee level as shown directly above.

EASIEST: Place the toes of your nonworking leg on the floor for added support and assistance.

Progressions

MAKE IT HARDER: Increase the range of motion so that your hips are lower than knee level.

EVEN HARDER: Employ an overhead arms progression by first crossing your arms and resting your hands on your shoulders (or holding your arms at chest level with your hands in prayer position). From there, place your hands behind your head (prisoner position). Next, fully extend both arms overhead.

HARDEST: Immediately follow a Single-Leg Wall Sit with a Double-Leg Wall Sit to fully fry your thighs beyond your wildest dreams. The other leg can provide just enough assistance to keep you going to further boost muscle growth and endurance.

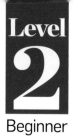

STEPUP

Stepups should be a staple of your lower-body training because going up and down stairs and stepping on and off curbs is a motion we perform every day and hope to do for a long lifetime. The Stepup is basically a reverse Single-Leg Squat with a much shorter learning curve—you start in the bottom of a Single-Leg Squat position with a little bit of support and assistance from your trailing leg. It's also one of the best butt-building exercises in existence and serves as a great diagnostic tool to assess your single-leg strength, stability, and balance. If you can't properly perform Stepups with a slow and controlled tempo through a pain-free full range of motion, then you have no business lunging, single-leg squatting, or running and jumping, for that matter.

How to Do It

Starting Position

● Place one foot on a sturdy box or step with your weight placed on the center of your foot (right in front of your anklebone).

● Establish tripod foot position for a natural foot arch with the knuckles of your big toe and little toe and your heel in contact with the ground.

● Your stepping leg should be elevated on a surface high enough that your knee is higher than your hip.

Perfect Execution

● First, push your hips back and then stand straight up, squeezing the glute of your supporting leg at the top of the movement.

● Hold this top position briefly while keeping your hips and shoulders square as your body fights the tilting and turning forces.

● Push your hips back again and slowly lower your trailing foot to the ground, taking at least 3 seconds on the way back down to the starting position.

Your Goal

You should be able to do multiple sets of 10 reps on each leg with your hip below knee level before moving to the next level.

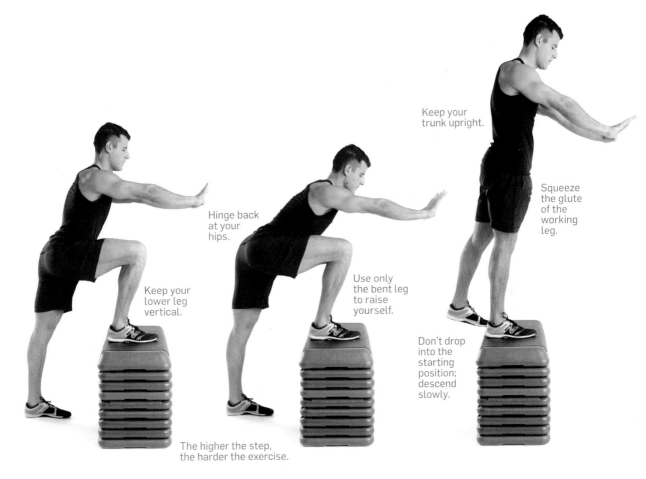

Keep your trunk upright.

Hinge back at your hips.

Keep your lower leg vertical.

Use only the bent leg to raise yourself.

Squeeze the glute of the working leg.

Don't drop into the starting position; descend slowly.

The higher the step, the harder the exercise.

Regressions

MAKE IT EASIER: Use a lower box or step.

EVEN EASIER: Place your hands on a wall or another stable object for assistance.

EASIEST: Perform a Stepup Hold with the foot of your trailing leg hovering just above the floor (or as close to the floor as you can get it based on the height of the step).

Progressions

MAKE IT HARDER: Do an overhead arms progression by crossing your arms and resting your hands on your shoulders (or holding your arms at chest level with your hands in prayer position). From there, place your hands behind your head (prisoner position). Next, fully extend both arms overhead.

EVEN HARDER: Perform Stepup Jumps, adding a jump at the top of each rep and landing softly into the starting position. You can perform all of your reps on the same leg or switch legs midair.

HARDEST: Perform Deep Stepups using a box high enough so that the hamstring of your working leg rests on top of your calf in the starting position. The higher the box, the more you need to hinge at your hips to properly execute the movement.

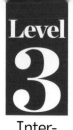

STAGGERED SQUAT

In sports you rarely use a perfectly parallel and symmetrical stance. More often your feet are staggered. That's why it's important to perform Squat variations with a staggered stance. Staggered Squats are a great stepping-stone exercise to the Single-Leg Squat plus they are easier on your back than regular Squats.

Special note: Understand the difference between a staggered stance and a split stance. A staggered stance has the toes of your trailing leg aligned with the heel of your leading leg and makes your quads and calves work harder. A split stance has the toes of your trailing leg placed farther behind your body (well past your hips) as if performing a stationary Lunge and makes your hips and hamstrings work harder. So a split stance is basically an extended staggered stance. It's best to start with Staggered Squats before progressing to Split Squats.

How to Do It

Starting Position

● Establish tripod foot position with your leading leg for a natural foot arch.

● With your feet hip-width apart, place the toes of your trailing leg on the floor so they are aligned with the heel of your leading leg.

● Keep most of your weight on the leading leg and treat the toes of the trailing leg like the kickstand of a bike that provides just enough support and assistance to stay upright.

Perfect Execution

● First, push your butt back and then sink your hips as low as you can until the hamstring of your leading leg rests on your calf.

● Hold this bottom position briefly and then stand up, being sure to fully extend your hips and squeeze your glutes at the top of the movement.

● Perform all of your reps on the same side before switching sides, always starting with your weak leg as the leading leg.

Your Goal

You should be able to do multiple sets of 10 reps on each leg with your hips below knee level before moving to the next level.

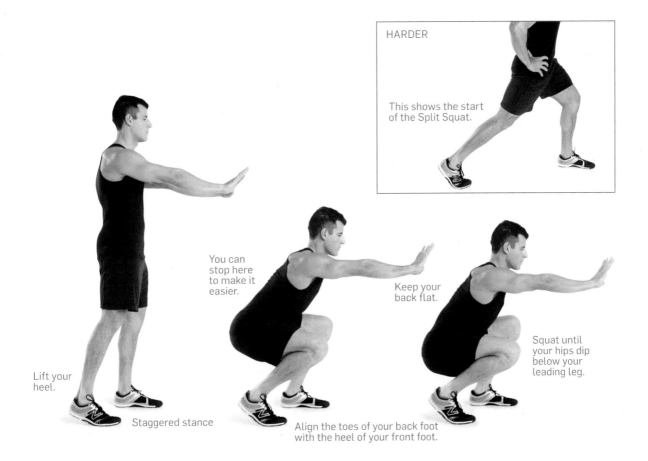

HARDER

This shows the start of the Split Squat.

You can stop here to make it easier.

Keep your back flat.

Squat until your hips dip below your leading leg.

Lift your heel.

Staggered stance

Align the toes of your back foot with the heel of your front foot.

Regressions

MAKE IT EASIER: Squat only to the point where your hip crease is slightly beneath your knee crease.

EVEN EASIER: Only squat as far as you can go in a pain-free range of motion.

EASIEST: Perform Self-Assisted Staggered Squats where your hands hold on to a TRX (or another suspension trainer) or a stable support system like a pole, railing, or ledge. This will allow you to use as much upper-body assistance as necessary to perform the movement pain free through a full range of motion.

Progressions

MAKE IT HARDER: Perform a Split Squat by moving from a staggered stance to a split stance. In the bottom position, there should be 90-degree angles at both knees and hips, with the knee of your trailing leg hovering just above the floor. Keep your torso fully upright, and squeeze the glute of your trailing leg and brace your core for full hip extension.

EVEN HARDER: Perform Rear-Foot-Elevated Split Squats (or Bulgarian Split Squats) by elevating your trailing leg on a stable box or chair at knee level. You can also elevate the trailing leg by securing it into the foot cradle of a suspension trainer to open up the hip flexor muscles of your trailing leg.

HARDEST: Perform a Front- and Rear-Foot-Elevated Split Squat by also elevating your front foot on a low box or weight plate.

LUNGE

Next to regular Squats, Lunges are probably the most popular bodyweight exercise for the lower body. But most people do them before they are ready for the challenge. Lunges are advanced exercises that require dynamic stability because you are changing the position of your feet and altering your base of support. Lots of Lunges will build wheels of steel, bulletproof your knees, and prepare your body for the demands of explosive movements like running and jumping. A longer Lunge step will make your hips and hamstrings work harder, whereas a shorter Lunge step will make your quads and calves work harder. Note that it's easier to perform all of your reps on one leg and then switch sides than it is to alternate legs every rep.

How to Do It

Starting Position

- Stand with your feet hip-width apart or closer.
- Establish tripod foot position for a natural foot arch.
- Keep your weight placed on the center of your foot (right in front of your ankle-bone) and your toes pointing straight ahead.

Perfect Execution

- Step back with one leg until your toes touch the ground, and then slowly pull your hips into the bottom of the Lunge.
- Hold this bottom position briefly with 90-degree angles at both knees and hips and with the knee of your trailing leg hovering just above the floor. There should be a straight line from the knee and hip of your trailing leg through your shoulders.
- Now pull your hips forward as you come back to full standing.

Your Goal

You should be able to do multiple sets of 10 reps on each leg before moving to the next level.

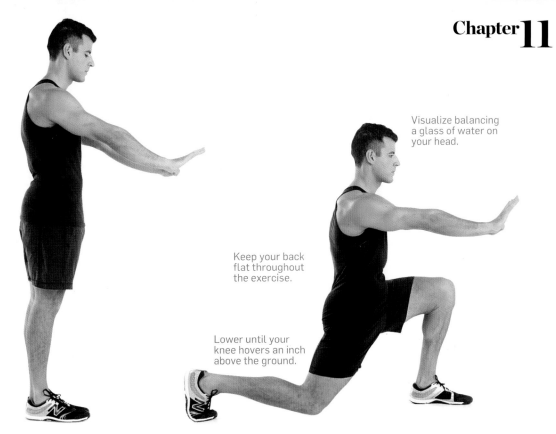

Visualize balancing a glass of water on your head.

Keep your back flat throughout the exercise.

Lower until your knee hovers an inch above the ground.

Regressions

MAKE IT EASIER: Lunge only as far as you can in a pain-free range of motion in a stepping manner.

EVEN EASIER: Take a smaller step backward to gain more stability and assistance from your trailing leg.

EASIEST: Perform Self-Assisted Lunges where your hands hold on to a suspension trainer or a stable support system like a pole, railing, or ledge. This will allow you to use as much upper-body assistance as necessary to perform the movement pain-free through a full range of motion.

Progressions

MAKE IT HARDER: Perform a Front-Foot-Elevated Reverse Lunge by placing your front foot on a low step or box to enhance the stretch.

EVEN HARDER: Perform Sliding Lunges by placing the foot of your back leg onto a Valslide, a towel, or a paper plate that will slide on a slick floor. Slide the foot back as you sink into the bottom position, then pull your hips forward to the starting position. Your back foot stays on the floor throughout.

HARDEST: Perform a Levitating Lunge. Lunge back until your knee, shin, and top of foot touch the ground (a). Progress further by lunging back until only your back knee touches and your leg is bent 90 degrees, foot off the floor (b).

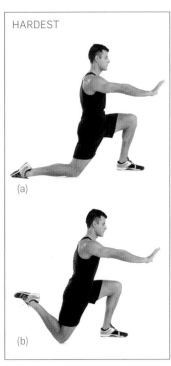

HARDEST

(a)

(b)

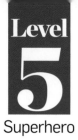

SINGLE-LEG SQUAT

It's important to note the difference between a Single-Leg Squat and a Pistol Squat. The former is any Squat on one leg to a depth where your hip crease is just above your knee crease. It doesn't matter what you do with your nonworking leg, though it is typically held behind your body, with your knee bent at a 90-degree angle. A Pistol Squat is a rock-bottom Squat on one leg where your working leg hamstring rests on your calf in the bottom position. The nonworking leg is fully extended in front of your body (requiring a great deal of hamstring flexibility), which is why your body resembles a pistol at the bottom of the move. Though your ultimate goal is to be able to gradually build up to a perfect Pistol Squat, keep in mind that this takes a lot of work, especially for larger and taller individuals. It also requires the hip and ankle mobility of a mutant and full pain-free flexion of the knee. That's why most people will do best with the Self-Assisted Pistol Squat variations or Pistol Box Squats on a low box or step. The bottom line is that a Single-Leg Squat provides 80 percent of the benefits of a perfect Pistol Squat, so don't sweat it if you feel like you're light-years away from the real deal.

How to Do It

Starting Position

- Stand on one leg and extend your other leg in front of your body.

- Establish tripod foot position. Keep your weight placed on the center of your foot (right in front of your anklebone).

- Hold a light weight with both hands for counter-balance with your arms extended in front of you.

Perfect Execution

- Push your hips and hamstrings back as far as you can (as if closing a door with your butt). Bend at the knee, and slowly lower yourself.

- Go as low as you can without overly rounding your lower back. If you can't get all the way down so that your hamstring rests on your calf, try to get at least low enough that your hip crease is slightly beneath your knee crease.

- Briefly pause in the bottom position and then extend your working leg and push your hips forward to come to full standing.

Your Goal

Once you can do multiple sets of 10 reps on each leg with your hips below knee level, you can call yourself a master of the Single-Leg Squat!

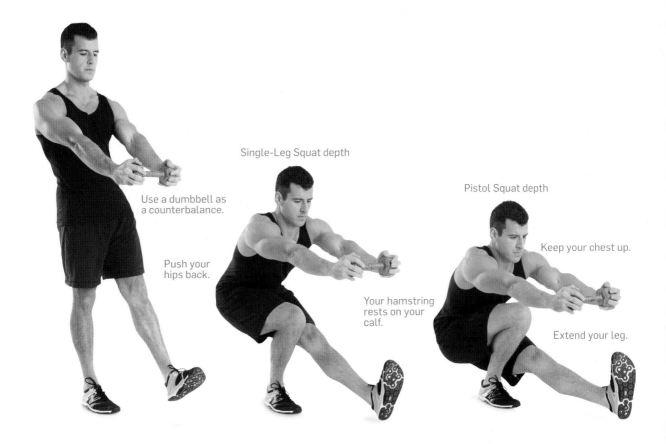

Single-Leg Squat depth

Use a dumbbell as a counterbalance.

Push your hips back.

Pistol Squat depth

Keep your chest up.

Your hamstring rests on your calf.

Extend your leg.

Regressions

MAKE IT EASIER: Perform a Single-Leg Box Squat where you sit down on a stable box. Your nonworking leg should be fully extended in front of your body as with a Pistol Squat. This variation fixes your form and makes you rely more on your hips and hamstrings to take pressure off of your knees. Progressively decrease the height of the box.

EVEN EASIER: Perform a Single-Leg Squat off a box with your working leg on a stable box. It's like a Deep Stepup with your nonworking leg dangling off to the side. Progressively increase the height of the box.

EASIEST: Perform Self-Assisted Single-Leg Squats where your hands hold on to a suspension trainer or a stable support. This will allow you to use as much upper-body assistance as necessary.

Progressions

MAKE IT HARDER: Eliminate the counterbalance by getting rid of the light weight held in your hands. This is one of the few times where less weight means greater difficulty.

EVEN HARDER: Do an overhead arms progression by crossing your arms with your hands resting on your shoulders (or holding your arms at chest level with your hands in prayer position). From there, place your hands behind your head (prisoner position). Next, fully extend both arms overhead.

HARDEST: Place your hands behind your body with the backs of your hands resting on the small of your lower back.

Variations

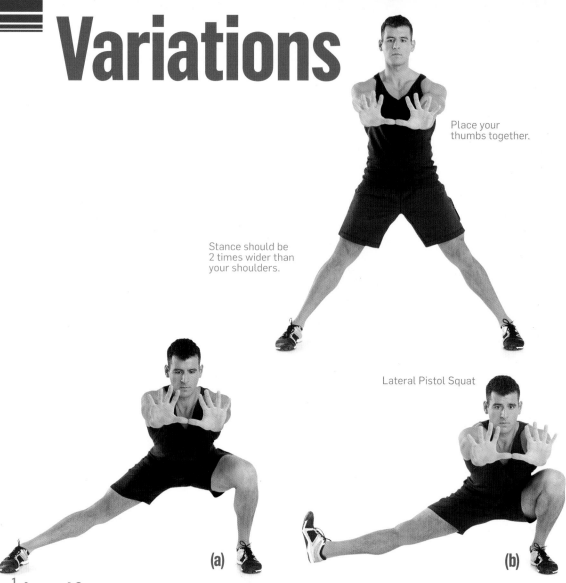

Place your thumbs together.

Stance should be 2 times wider than your shoulders.

Lateral Pistol Squat

(a)

(b)

1. Lateral Squat

Start with a superwide stance with your feet wider than shoulder-width apart and your toes pointing straight ahead. First, push your butt back and then to the side as you sink your hips down and shift your weight to your leading leg (a). The ideal range of motion has the hamstring resting on the calf of the working leg as if in the bottom of a Pistol Squat,

which is why I tend to call it a Lateral Pistol Squat (b). However, you can modify the motion by sinking down only to the point where your hip crease is slightly beneath your knee crease. Notice how the toes of your trailing leg point upward when you reach the bottom position. Keep your hips and shoulders square throughout the movement.

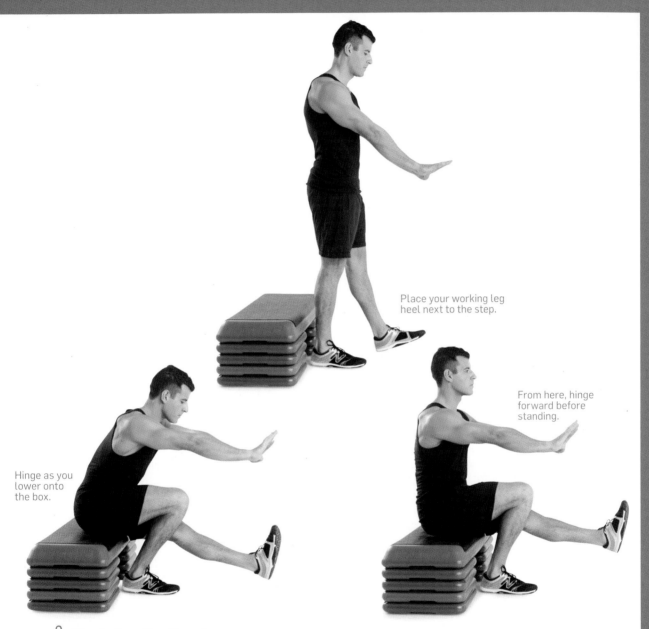

Place your working leg heel next to the step.

From here, hinge forward before standing.

Hinge as you lower onto the box.

2. Single-Leg Box Squat

Sit on a stable box while on one leg. Your nonworking leg should be fully extended in front of your body as with a Pistol Squat. This variation fixes your form and makes you rely more on your hips and hamstrings to get the job done to take pressure off of your knees. Progressively decrease the height of the box until it's only a couple inches off of the floor or you achieve full Pistol Squat range of motion.

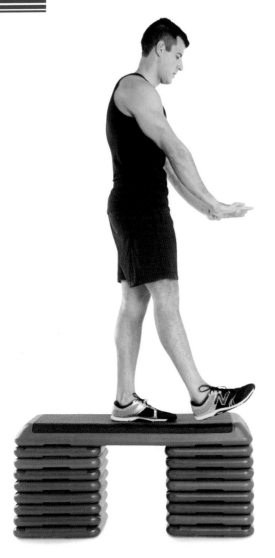

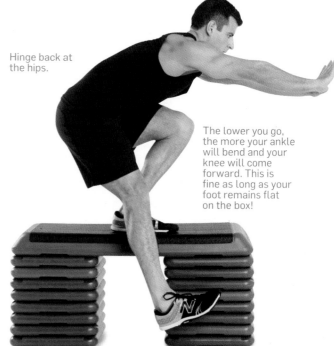

Hinge back at the hips.

The lower you go, the more your ankle will bend and your knee will come forward. This is fine as long as your foot remains flat on the box!

3. Single-Leg Squat off Box

Stand on a high box or step while on one leg. Hinge your hips and bend your knee until your working leg thigh is almost parallel to the floor. This setup is easier than a Pistol Squat because you don't need the hamstring flexibility and hip flexor strength to extend the nonworking leg in front of your body. Increase the height of the box until you can get full depth without letting the foot of your nonworking leg touch the floor.

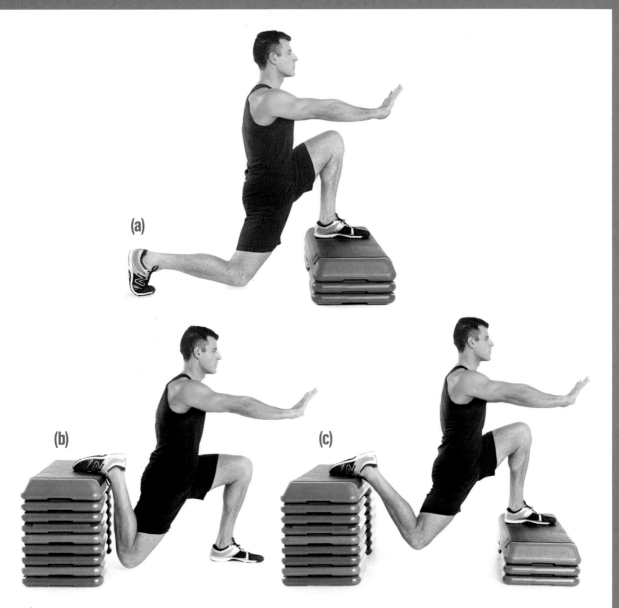

(a)

(b)

(c)

4. Extended Range of Motion Split Squat Series

First, perform Front-Foot-Elevated Split Squats (a) by elevating your front foot on a low box or step. Then, progress to Rear-Foot-Elevated Split Squats (or Bulgarian Split Squats[b]) by elevating your back leg on a stable box, step, or chair at or just below knee level. You can also elevate the trailing leg by securing it into the foot cradle of a suspension trainer. Finally, combine both options (c). This will allow your hips to sink as deep as they do with a Staggered Squat, with the added difficulty of a split stance.

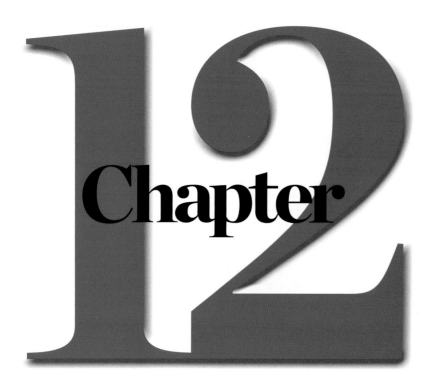

Chapter 12

BODYWEIGHT 8: PULLUP

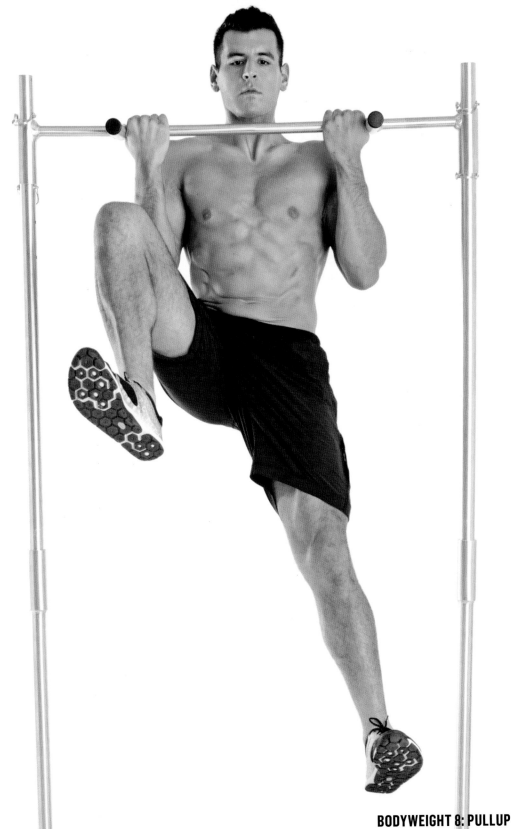

#8
PULLUP

The Pullup is the best exercise to shape a classic V-tapered torso. It's also one of the most primal. The ability to pull the body up into trees to evade predators was vital to human survival. Today, few tasks require us to pull our own body weight, and, as a result, our back muscles have become weak. Plenty of things we do require us to push with our hands, like pushing ourselves out of bed or up from a car seat. All this pushing with little pulling results in poor grip strength and a pathetic posture—head forward, shoulders rounded, hunched back—that leads to shoulder injuries.

Pullups will forge strong shoulders, forearms, and hands to give you the functional strength of a professional mover and a handshake that shows people you mean business. Most important, hanging vertically provides much-needed spinal decompression that lubricates your intervertebral disks. Like hitting a Handstand or a Deep Squat, hanging from a bar for as long as you can once a day is a guaranteed way to make you feel and move better right away.

As with the Row, the Pullup requires something from which to hang. Best options include a freestanding Pullup unit, a door Pullup bar, or a TRX suspension trainer (or pair of gymnastics rings) that is vertically anchored to a sturdy rafter, tree branch, or power rack. If you don't want to spend money on equipment, you have several alternatives at home or in a hotel room. One, you can hold on to the top of a sturdy door with an overhand grip. (Place a towel or book underneath the door to unload the hinges.) It will feel better on your hands and fingers to wrap a thick towel over the top of the door before you grab it. Door Pullups are actually a bit harder than regular Pullups because of the friction between your body and the door as you go up and down. In addition, they keep your elbows closer to your body and prevent you from cheating because you can't swing your body back and forth. A tree branch, ledge, or horizontal bar at a playground makes for good Pullup opportunities. If none of these options works for you, there are equipment-free substitutes at the end of this chapter.

The PULLUP Progression

Level 1	Level 2	Level 3	Level 4	Level 5
Ground Zero	Beginner	Intermediate	Advanced	Superhero
DEAD HANG	FLEXED HANG	ECCENTRIC PULLUP	PULLUP	SELF-ASSISTED SINGLE-ARM PULLUP

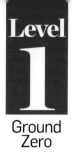
DEAD HANG

You can't do a Pullup if you can't Dead Hang, so this is the place to start. Hang from the bar in a hollow-body position with your legs fully extended and slightly in front of your body instead of having your legs bent behind your body as most people do. Legs extended makes it easier to brace your core and squeeze your glutes to prevent your lower back from hyperextending during the movement. If you can't find a high-enough apparatus to hang from so that your legs can fully extend without touching the floor, just move your legs farther in front of your body. Or bend your knees in front of you. This is still a stronger core position than bending them behind you. Remember, the Dead Hang is a hanging Plank, so it's all about keeping your ribs and shoulders down, squeezing your glutes, and bracing your core.

As with Rows, I suggest using a hook grip. Wrap your fingers over the top of the bar and your thumb under. From there, clasp your thumb around your index and/or middle finger. Flex your wrists slightly so that your pinkie finger will slide over the top of the bar. This is your strongest gripping position. It stabilizes your shoulders by creating an external rotation force that screws them into the sockets.

How to Do It

Starting Position

• Grab the bar or handles of a suspension trainer with a hook grip.

• Set your head in a neutral position with your ears aligned with your shoulders, hips, and ankles, and keep your gaze centered between your hands.

• Assume a hollow-body position with your legs straight and your toes pointing away from your body: Squeeze your legs together, tense your thighs, clench your glutes, brace your abs, and pull your ribs and shoulders down.

Perfect Execution

• Hold this Dead Hang position for time while actively maintaining hollow-body mechanics for the duration of the exercise.

• Focus on deep belly breathing to prevent your ribs from rising.

Your Goal

You should be able to do multiple sets of 60-second holds before moving to the next level.

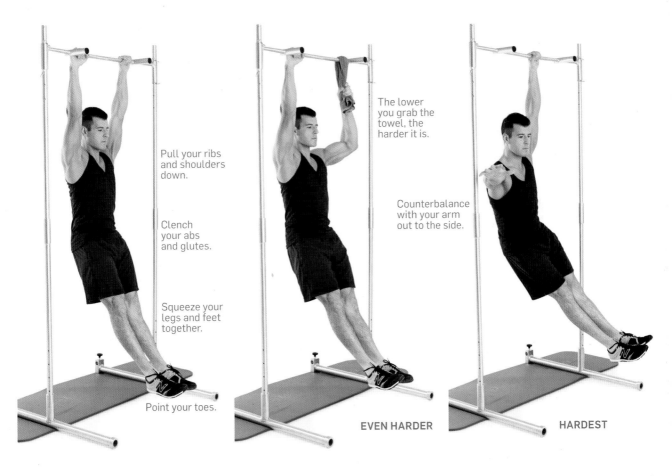

Pull your ribs and shoulders down.

Clench your abs and glutes.

Squeeze your legs and feet together.

Point your toes.

The lower you grab the towel, the harder it is.

Counterbalance with your arm out to the side.

EVEN HARDER

HARDEST

Regressions

MAKE IT EASIER: Perform Self-Assisted Dead Hangs by placing your toes on the floor. You'll need to hang from something stable that allows you to keep your arms fully extended.

EVEN EASIER: Add more self-assistance by placing your feet flat on the floor, not just your toes.

EASIEST: If you still find the previous regressions too challenging, simply perform a Hanging Bridge as outlined in Chapter 8. A horizontal Hang is easier than a vertical Hang because you're supporting less of your total body weight.

Progressions

MAKE IT HARDER: Perform a Close-Grip Dead Hang. Progressively bring your hands closer together until your thumbs touch.

EVEN HARDER: Perform an Uneven-Grip Dead Hang. Place a thick towel or rope around the bar or handle and hold the towel ends in the assisting hand. The lower you grab on the towel with your assisting arm, the harder the other arm will have to work.

HARDEST: Perform Single-Arm Dead Hangs. Place the hand of your working arm directly above your same-side shoulder. Move your nonworking arm behind your back or out to the side for extra counterbalance.

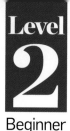

FLEXED HANG

The Flexed Hang adds a bend to your elbows, making it harder to hang from that position. Your first goal is to be able to perform a Flexed Hang in the midrange of a Pullup position with your elbows bent at 90-degree angles (a). Your next goal is to do a fully Flexed Hang with your elbows fully bent (b) and your body in the top of the Pullup position with your chest as close to the bar as possible. *Note:* If you have longer arms (particularly forearms), your chest probably won't touch the bar even if your elbows and shoulders go through a full range of motion. Just focus on getting your elbows close to your ribs without shrugging your shoulders or driving your head forward.

I like to say that if you can own the tops and bottoms of a given movement, you will own everything in between. The Dead Hang prepared you for the starting position of a Pullup; the Flexed Hang prepares you for the finish. These isometric holds will help you build the strength to perform full-range-of-motion reps of Pullups.

How to Do It

Starting Position

- Grab the bar or handles of a suspension trainer with a hook grip.

- Set your head in a neutral position with your ears aligned with your shoulders, hips, and ankles, and look between your hands.

- Assume a hollow-body position with your legs straight and your toes pointing away from your body: Squeeze your legs together, tense your glutes and abs, and pull your ribs and shoulders down.

Perfect Execution

- Cheat yourself into the top of the Pullup position by either jumping up or stepping from a sturdy chair, step, or bench. Use your legs to assist your upper body.

- Hold this Flexed Hang position for time while actively maintaining hollow-body mechanics for the duration of the exercise.

- Focus on deep belly breathing to prevent your ribs from rising.

Your Goal

You should be able to do multiple sets of 30-second holds before moving to the next level.

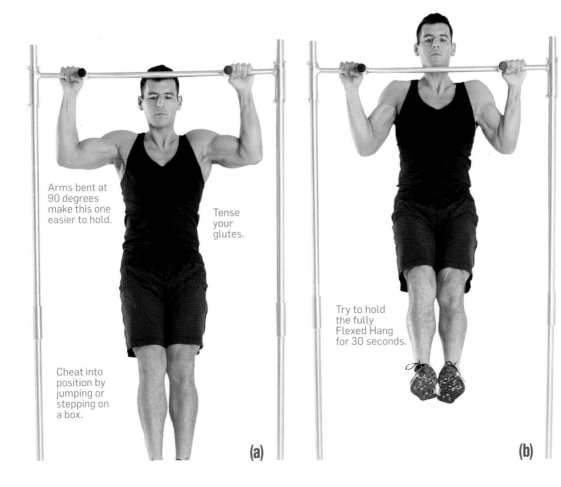

Arms bent at 90 degrees make this one easier to hold.

Tense your glutes.

Cheat into position by jumping or stepping on a box.

Try to hold the fully Flexed Hang for 30 seconds.

(a)

(b)

Regressions

MAKE IT EASIER: Minimize the range of motion by performing a Flexed Hang with your elbows bent at 90-degree angles (a). You can also break up longer holds into shorter 5- to 10-second holds with 2- to 5-second breaks between holds.

EVEN EASIER: Use a neutral grip with your palms facing each other. This variation emphasizes your forearms.

EASIEST: Use an underhand grip with your palms facing your body. This move is an unmatched biceps builder.

Progressions

MAKE IT HARDER: Perform Close-Grip Flexed Hangs. Bring your hands closer together until your thumbs touch.

EVEN HARDER: Perform Uneven-Grip Flexed Hangs. Place a thick towel or rope around the bar or handle and hold the towel ends in the assisting hand. The lower you grab on the towel with your assisting arm, the harder the other arm will have to work.

HARDEST: Perform Single-Arm Flexed Hangs. Place the hand of your working arm directly above your same-side shoulder. These are extremely challenging, and even the most advanced trainees will still need to use some self-assistance.

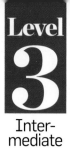

3

Inter-
mediate

ECCENTRIC PULLUP

Practicing the second half of a Pullup will help you master the first. Your muscles are stronger during the eccentric (or lowering) phase of an exercise when they are lengthening as opposed to the concentric (or lifting) phase when they are shortening. Eccentric Pullups allow you to focus on the lowering portion of the exercise to build up the strength you need to eventually be able to pull yourself up without assistance. You can apply eccentric-only emphasis to any advanced movement in this book as long as you take at least 3 to 5 seconds to smoothly perform the lowering portion of that movement.

How to Do It

Starting Position

● Grab the bar or handles of a suspension trainer with a hook grip.

● Set your head in a neutral position with your ears aligned with your shoulders, hips, and ankles, and keep your gaze centered between your hands.

● Assume a hollow-body position with your legs straight and your toes pointing away from your body: Squeeze your legs together, tense your thighs, clench your glutes, brace your abs, and pull your ribs and shoulders down.

Perfect Execution

● Cheat yourself into the top of the Pullup position by either jumping up or stepping from a stable chair, step, box, or bench. The goal is to use your legs to assist your upper body.

● Then slowly lower your body to a Dead Hang, taking at least 3 to 5 seconds to do so while maintaining hollow-body mechanics during the descent.

● Cheat back up again and repeat.

Your Goal

You should be able to do multiple sets of 10 reps before moving to the next level.

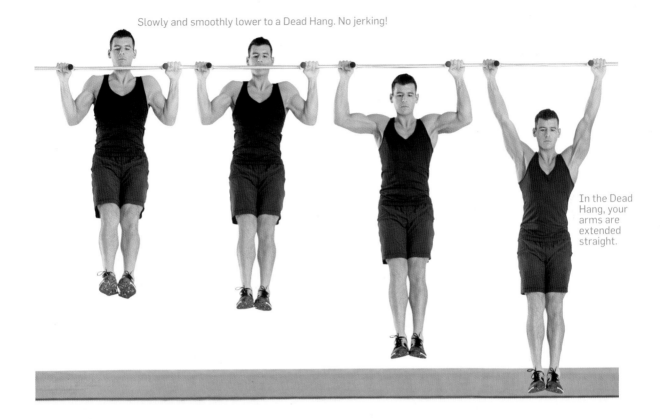

Slowly and smoothly lower to a Dead Hang. No jerking!

In the Dead Hang, your arms are extended straight.

Regressions

MAKE IT EASIER: Shorten the lowering time to 1 or 2 seconds or as slowly as you can do it with control.

EVEN EASIER: Use a neutral grip with your palms facing each other. This variation emphasizes your forearms.

EASIEST: Use an underhand grip with your palms facing your body. This move is an unmatched biceps builder.

Progressions

MAKE IT HARDER: Lengthen the lowering time to 6 to 10 seconds or more.

EVEN HARDER: Perform Close-Grip Eccentric Pullups. Bring your hands closer together until your thumbs touch. You can also make it harder on your shoulders by placing your hands wider than shoulder-width apart.

HARDEST: Perform Uneven-Grip Eccentric Pullups. Place a thick towel or rope around the bar and hold the towel ends in the assisting hand. The lower you grab on the towel, the greater the mechanical disadvantage to that arm, making it harder on your working arm.

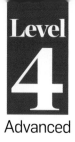

Level

4

Advanced

PULLUP

The Pullup is the exact opposite movement pattern of the Handstand Pushup, making them perfect exercises to superset, or alternate between. A good rule of thumb is to perform at least as many total sets/reps for Pullups as you do for Handstand Pushups. If you have a history of shoulder pain, poor posture, or doing lots of overhead pressing, then do two to three times as many sets/reps for Pullups as for Handstand Pushups to correct this structural imbalance. Pullups are all about persistence, and many people need to get over the mental block that comes with never having been able to do them before. You can do it; you'll see.

You can perform Pullups using many different grips. A normal grip is overhand with your hands about shoulder-width apart. You can go wider to make your upper back and rear shoulders work harder or closer to emphasize your forearms and biceps. Use an underhand grip to shift the work more to your biceps. Many pullup bars have a neutral-grip option where your palms face each other. Using a suspension trainer allows you to rotate your hands as you pull, which tends to be easier on the shoulders.

How to Do It

Starting Position

• Grab the bar or handles of a suspension trainer with a hook grip.

• Set your head in a neutral position with your ears aligned with your shoulders, hips, and ankles, and look between your hands.

• Assume a hollow-body position with your legs straight and your toes pointing away from your body: Squeeze your legs together, tense your thighs, glutes, and abs, and pull your ribs and shoulders down.

Perfect Execution

• Pull yourself up from a Dead Hang until your elbows reach your ribs and your chest is as close to the bar as you can get without shrugging your shoulders or driving your head forward. Don't worry about getting your chin over the bar!

• Hold this position for 1 or 2 seconds, then slowly lower your body back to a Dead Hang while maintaining hollow-body mechanics throughout the movement.

Your Goal

You should ideally be able to perform multiple sets of 10 reps before progressing to the next level.

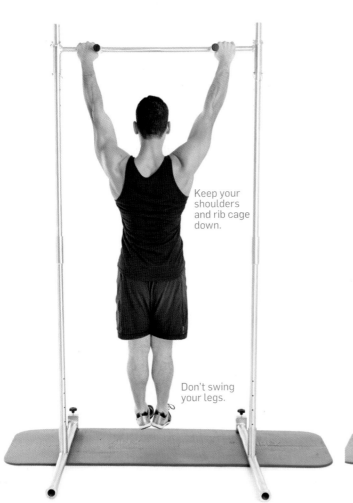

Keep your shoulders and rib cage down.

Don't swing your legs.

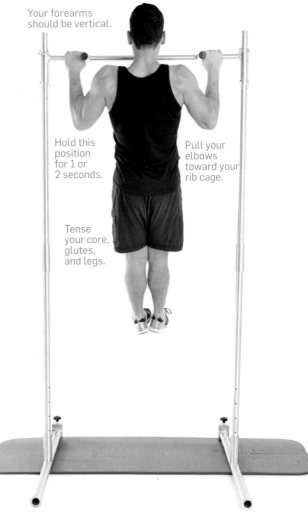

Your forearms should be vertical.

Hold this position for 1 or 2 seconds.

Pull your elbows toward your rib cage.

Tense your core, glutes, and legs.

Regressions

MAKE IT EASIER: Shift to a neutral grip with your palms facing each other.

EVEN EASIER: Use an underhand grip with your palms facing your body.

EASIEST: Perform Self-Assisted Pullups by keeping your feet on the floor and using your legs for assistance. Start by only using one leg for assistance. If you need more help, use both legs.

Progressions

MAKE IT HARDER: Increase the range of motion by performing Close-Grip Pullups. Bring your hands closer together until your thumbs touch.

EVEN HARDER: Shift the work to your upper back, lats, and rear shoulders with Wide-Grip Pullups. Place your hands wider than shoulder-width apart.

HARDEST: Perform $1\frac{1}{2}$ Pullups. Pull yourself up, but then lower yourself only halfway down until your upper arms are parallel to the floor. Then pull yourself all the way back up again and finally lower all the way down to a Dead Hang. That's 1 rep. Repeat.

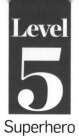
SELF-ASSISTED SINGLE-ARM PULLUP

This is another "tweener" exercise to ease you into a true Single-Arm Pullup. Here, one arm does 70 percent or more of the lifting. The best place to start is with Staggered Pullups. The hand of the working arm should grab the pullup bar or handle as normal. Wrap a towel around the bar for your assisting hand. This shifts more of the load onto your working arm. Make sure to keep your hips and shoulders square to the ground.

How to Do It

Starting Position

● Grab the bar/handle with your working arm just above your shoulder as usual. Wrap a towel around the bar and grab both ends with your assisting hand.

● Set your head in a neutral position with your ears aligned with your shoulders, hips, and ankles, and look between your hands.

● Assume a hollow-body position with your legs straight and your toes pointing away from your body: Squeeze your legs together, tense your thighs, clench your glutes, brace your abs, and pull your ribs and shoulders down.

Perfect Execution

● Pull yourself up from a Dead Hang until your elbows reach your ribs and your chest is as close to the bar as you can get without shrugging your shoulders. Don't worry about getting your chin over the bar!

● Hold this position for 1 or 2 seconds, then slowly lower your body back to a Dead Hang while maintaining hollow-body position.

Your Goal

You should ideally be able to perform multiple sets of 10 reps per side.

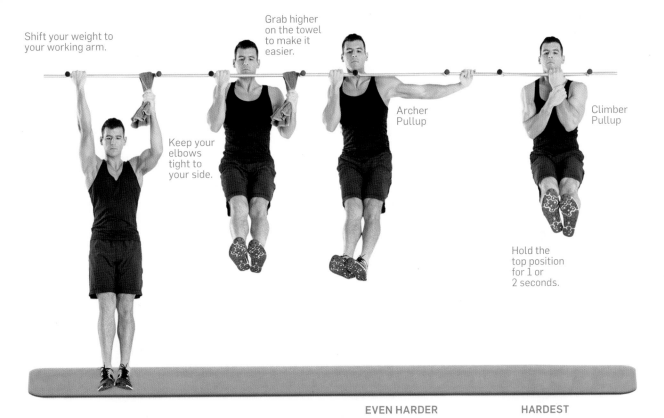

Shift your weight to your working arm.

Grab higher on the towel to make it easier.

Keep your elbows tight to your side.

Archer Pullup

Climber Pullup

Hold the top position for 1 or 2 seconds.

EVEN HARDER   HARDEST

Regressions

MAKE IT EASIER: Shift to neutral grip with the palm of your working arm facing inward.

EVEN EASIER: Use an underhand grip with the palm of your working arm facing your body.

EASIEST: Perform Single-Arm Squat Pullups. Hold on to a pullup bar that's set low enough so that your feet touch the ground and you can sink all the way down into the Deep Squat position. You can also hold on to the handles of a TRX or another suspension trainer that's vertically anchored above you. Pull up with one arm, using only as much assistance as you need from both legs. Progress by performing Single-Arm, Single-Leg Squat Pullups with only one leg providing assistance. You can use your arms and legs equally for more of a total-body fat-loss exercise or choose to use mostly your arms for more of an upper-body muscle builder.

Progressions

MAKE IT HARDER: Use less self-assistance by grabbing lower on the towel.

EVEN HARDER: Use less self-assistance and decrease your leverage with Archer Pullups. Fully extend the arm of your assisting hand directly to the side. You can also progressively place fewer fingertips on the bar until only one or two fingers remain.

HARDEST: Perform Climber Pullups, also known as One-Handed Pullups. Inspired by the gripping work of rock climbers, this is the most advanced Self-Assisted Single-Arm Pullup option because one hand is supporting your entire body. Grab the bar or handle with your working arm. Then grab the wrist of your working arm with your assisting hand. Pull your body up using only as much assistance as you need from the assisting hand. Make it harder by moving the assisting hand lower on your arm.

Variations

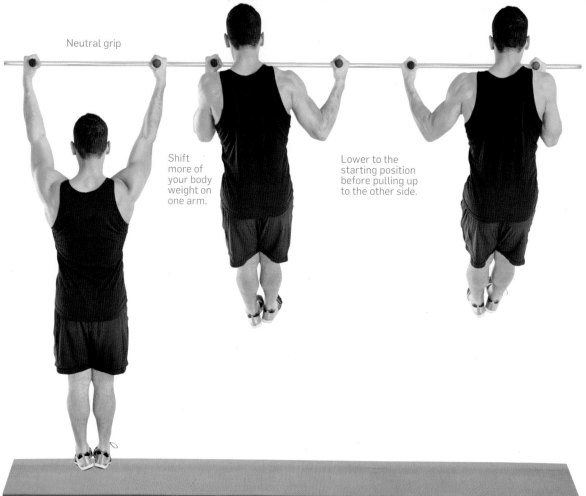

Neutral grip

Shift more of your body weight on one arm.

Lower to the starting position before pulling up to the other side.

1. Side-to-Side Pullup

Begin this exercise like a normal two-arm Pullup, but as you pull your body upward, slowly shift your weight as much to one side as you can. Then lower back to the starting position. You can either switch sides every rep or perform all of your reps on one side before switching. Make this harder by starting with your hands a bit wider apart to make your leading arm pull more of your body weight.

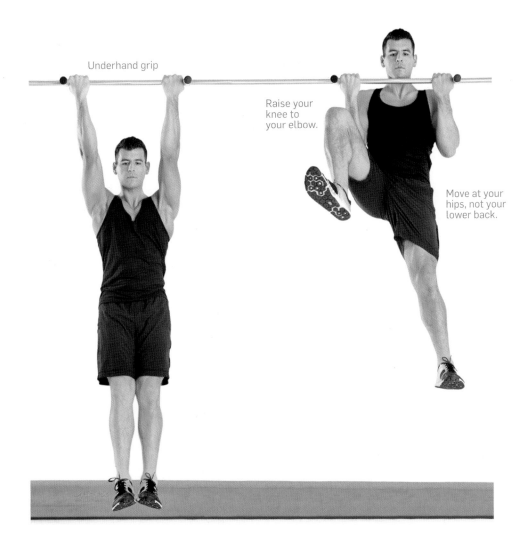

Underhand grip

Raise your knee to your elbow.

Move at your hips, not your lower back.

2. Spider Pullup

Another way to shift more work to one side of your body during Pullups is to add leg movement. A Spider Pullup has you flex your hip and bring one knee to the same-side elbow as you pull your body up. You can make it harder by fully extending that same leg to the side once you reach the top position. This forces you to shift more weight to the opposite arm for counterbalance. You can either perform all of your reps on one side before switching or switch sides every rep.

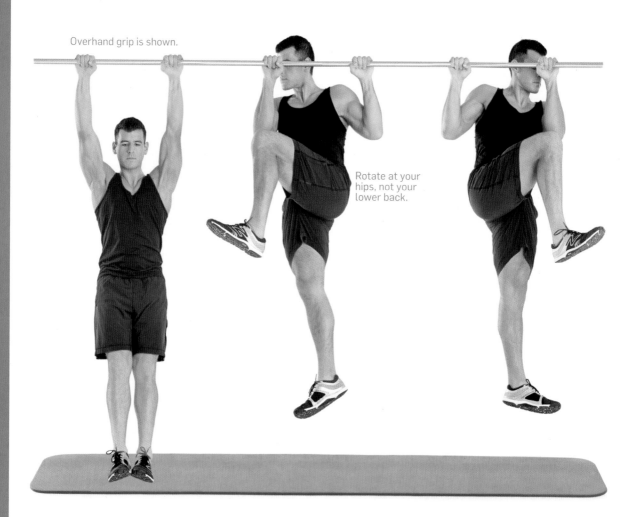

Overhand grip is shown.

Rotate at your hips, not your lower back.

3. Cross-Body Pullup

This is very similar to a Spider Pullup, except that you rotate your hips to bring a knee to the opposite elbow as you pull yourself up. Note that you will not be able to do this exercise with as much range of motion as a normal Pullup. This is a killer core exercise.

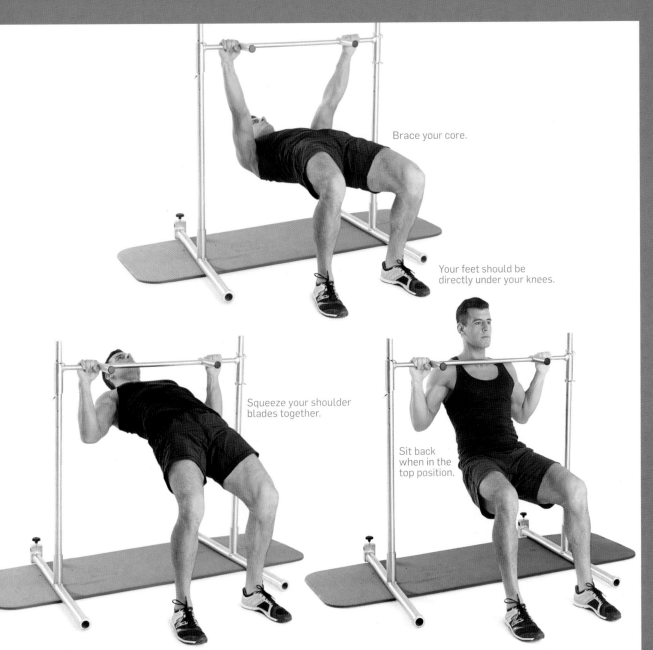

Brace your core.

Your feet should be directly under your knees.

Squeeze your shoulder blades together.

Sit back when in the top position.

4. Row to Pullup

This is a great stepping-stone exercise to a regular Pullup. It also works all of your upper-body pulling muscles from every angle in between a horizontal pull (Row) and a vertical pull (Pullup). With your feet on the floor, perform a Row and then sit your hips back until you end up with a vertical body position at the top of a Pullup. Reverse the movement and repeat.

Equipment-Free Pullup Options

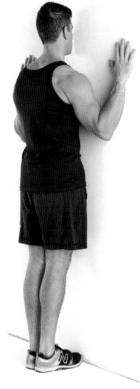

Press against the wall to create friction resistance.

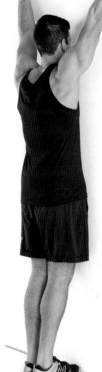

Keep your armpits forward.

1. Wall Slide

This is a great warmup/corrective exercise or a substitute for Pullups if you are unable to find something to hang from. It can be performed either facing or facing away from a wall or closed door. For the facing version, stand right in front of a wall with your toes touching the wall. Place your hands and forearms on the wall and then slowly slide them up the wall until your arms are fully extended without allowing your ribs or shoulders to rise or your lower back to overly arch. Reverse the movement and repeat. For the facing-away version, place your heels, head, upper back, and butt against the wall. Slowly slide your arms up and down. For both versions, you're trying to mimic the Pullup motion and use the wall to create enough friction to provide some tension to your upper-back/midback muscles.

2. Band Pulldown

Wrap a single resistance band around an overhead bar or other anchor point and hold one end in each hand. If the anchor point isn't high enough to achieve enough resistance or get enough range of motion, simply get on your knees. Pull the band to your armpits with the same form cues as a Pullup, reverse the movement, and repeat. Make it harder by grabbing higher up on the band or by using a thicker band.

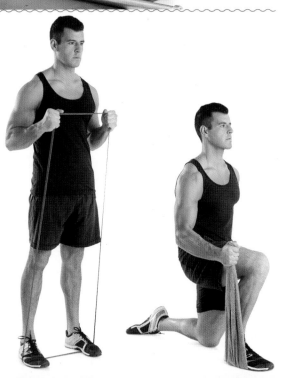

3. Band Curl and Iso Towel Curl

Stand on a resistance band and grab the ends in each hand. Keeping your elbows tight to your sides and your shoulders down and back, flex your elbows and raise your hands to as close to your shoulders as you can. Reverse the movement and repeat. If you don't have bands, you can use a towel. Step on one end of a towel and kneel on the other leg. Hold the other end of the towel in one hand so your elbow is bent at 90 degrees with your forearm parallel to the floor. Pull on the towel as hard as you can and hold for time. You can also stand on the middle of a beach towel and exercise both arms at the same time.

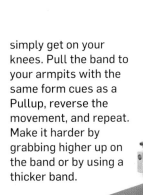

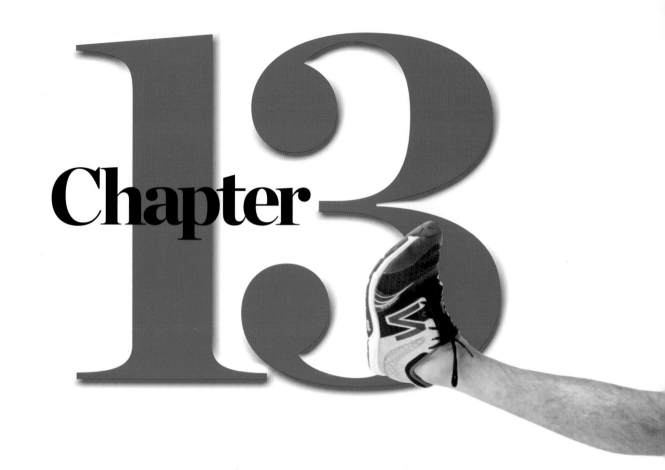

Chapter 13

BODYWEIGHT BURNERS PROGRAM

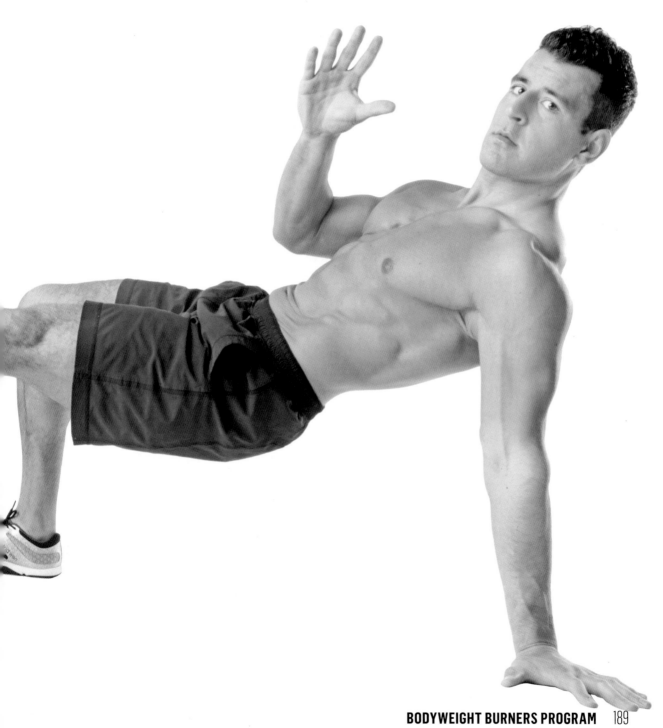

You now have eight amazing exercise moves in your fat-torching arsenal. These are so effective and versatile that they're really the only eight exercises you need to master to get into great shape with just your body weight. Now it's time to show you how to combine these exercises into body-changing workouts that you can do anytime, anywhere.

The bodyweight programs that follow in this chapter and the next were choreographed with two types of exercisers in mind: rigid exercisers and flexible exercisers. Rigid exercisers prefer very structured programs that set out exactly what to do from start to finish. No guesswork, just results. Flexible exercisers prefer to take ownership of their programs; they thrive on constant variety and a feeling of control. They tend to do better by working within a bunch of workout templates that let them customize their workouts to their specific goals.

Most beginners prefer the rigid approach because they like a lot of guidance and it helps them to have a set training schedule. But as beginners progress and get leaner, stronger, and more confident, they tend to want to try new things, and they become more flexible in their workouts. I've known a lot of fitness professionals who started out as overweight and out-of-shape beginners. After transforming their bodies—and ultimately their lives—they go all in and eventually follow a career path of changing the bodies and lives of others. Heck, I'm one of them!

So we'll begin with beginners in mind, using a rigid-style workout called the Bodyweight Burners Program. It's a five-phase program designed to take you from ground zero to superhero, and it's ideal for the exerciser who wants some structure. This program is perfect for you if:

❶ You have a lot of body fat to lose.

❷ You are new to bodyweight training.

❸ You are looking for a jump-start to get back in shape.

In the next chapter, you'll find the Bodyweight 8 workouts for the flexible exerciser, which include my favorite bodyweight training templates that you can mix and match at your pleasure. These workouts are best for people who:

❶ Are already exercising regularly.

❷ Have greater fitness knowledge.

❸ Have already completed the Bodyweight Burners Program.

It's time to make a change, baby!

THE BODYWEIGHT BURNERS PROGRAM

This is the simplest and most effective rapid-fat-loss program you'll find anywhere using nothing but your body weight. The high-intensity 60-second work periods burn the sugar stored in your muscles, which shifts your body into a turbocharged fat-burning state during rest periods and in the hours and days between workouts. The short, incomplete 15-second rest periods give you just enough time to recover and transition to the next exercise, which maximizes key fat-burning hormones like growth hormone and keeps your heart rate elevated throughout the workout to improve your cardio conditioning and boost calorie-burning. Studies show that this type of metabolic resistance-training circuit can elevate your metabolism for 48 hours or more after completing your workout. Depending on your body size, fitness level, and gender, you can expect to burn 20 calories or more every minute.

There are five phases in this program, each phase lasting 28 days, or 4 weeks, for 5 months total. This is a progressive program: Each phase is matched with the appropriate exercise level for each Bodyweight 8 exercise. In Phase 1, you'll be using all of the Level 1 exercise variations; in Phase 2, you'll be using the Level 2 exercise variations; and so forth. You can expect to see significant results within the first 28 days—specifically, 10 or more pounds of weight loss, stronger muscles, and increased energy. What's more, you'll sleep better, your mood will improve, and you'll reap countless health benefits. And by the end of this 5-month total-body transformation program, you will be a lean, mean fitness machine! What does that mean exactly? You can reasonably expect to lower your body-fat percentage into the teens and be in the best shape of your life—I'm talking about fitness-model shape with well-defined lean muscle and abs that ripple.

Here's how it works.

Perform this whole-body workout three times per week with ideally 48 hours between workouts. For example, perform these workouts on Mondays, Wednesdays, and Fridays.

Alternate between 60 seconds of work and 15 seconds of rest for each exercise in the bodyweight circuit. Here's the general order of exercises.

1. Hip Thrust Variation
2. Pushup Variation
3. Deep Squat Variation
4. Row Variation
5. Hip Hinge Variation
6. Handstand Pushup Variation
7. Single-Leg Squat Variation
8. Pullup Variation

Each circuit is 10 minutes in duration. For best results, I recommend that you perform at least three total cycles for a 30-minute workout. If you're short on time or just getting back into shape, perform one or two cycles for a 10- or 20-minute workout. If you have more time to train or already train regularly, perform four to six cycles for a 40- to 60-minute workout. This is your program, so feel free to customize it to your exact schedule and fitness level.

Perform as many quality reps as you can with perfect form and technique within each 60-second work period. If it's an isometric exercise, simply hold the position for as long as you can. If you need to rest, pause at any point during a given work period and resume when ready before time is up. This is referred to as rest-pause training and it allows you to do more overall reps with a harder exercise variation (or a heavier load) over multiple sets using short 5- to 20-second rest periods than you could accomplish with a single set. This leads to greater strength and muscle gains and enhanced fat loss. In a recent study published in the *Journal of Translational Medicine*, experienced lifters burned 18 percent more calories 22 hours after using the rest-pause workout technique than they burned after doing a traditional single-set workout. What's more, the lifters lost more body fat. Your ultimate goal is to eventually be able to work continuously for the full 60 seconds without stopping.

For all unilateral exercises (where you use one limb at a time), be sure to switch sides at the halfway mark so you perform 30 seconds of work on each side, always starting with your weak side first when you're most fresh. You could also perform all your reps/work on one side for the full minute and then switch sides from cycle to cycle, if you'd like. Just make sure to perform an equal number of sets/reps on each side and an even number of total cycles of the circuit (two, four, or six instead of three). A final option is to perform a single rep on one side, then switch sides, and keep alternating for 1 minute. I like this for really challenging moves like Pistol Squats, Single-Arm Pushups, and Self-Assisted Single-Arm Pullups because it keeps the intensity high and ensures that you're not too fatigued before you switch sides. You also don't have to worry about looking at a clock to figure out when to switch sides.

In general, you should be able to perform at least 10 total reps (5 per side for a unilateral movement) within each 60-second work

Level 1
Ground Zero (28 Days)

1
HIP THRUST
(page 48)

2
PLANK
(page 66)

3
WALL SIT
(page 84)

4
HANGING BRIDGE
(page 100)

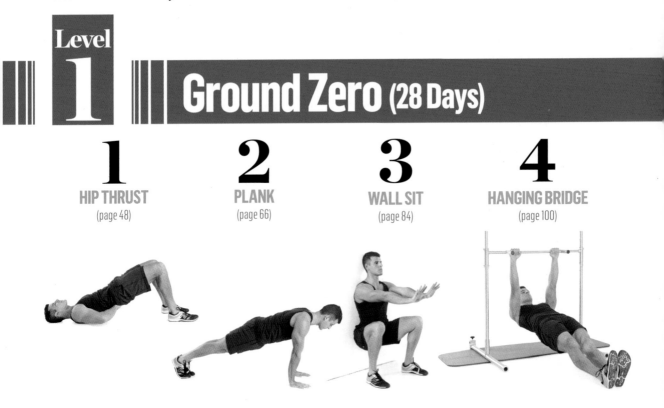

period. If you're consistently getting fewer than 10 total reps, make the exercise easier by using one of the microregressions within each exercise level. If you're consistently getting more than 10 total reps, make the exercise harder by using one of the microprogressions within each exercise level.

If you're using plyometric exercises like Squat Jumps, Vertical Jumps, Plyo Pushups, or Plyo Rows, pause for 4 to 5 seconds in the top or bottom position between explosive reps to emphasize quality over quantity. You can also alternate between 10 seconds of work and 10 seconds of rest three times to fill the full minute. Just don't do fast jumping movements for a minute straight; the risk of injury is greater than the reward.

After 28 days (4 weeks), move up to the next exercise level in the program.

Month 1: Level 1 Ground Zero
Month 2: Level 2 Beginner
Month 3: Level 3 Intermediate
Month 4: Level 4 Advanced
Month 5: Level 5 Superhero

You can also employ the drop-set technique for some additional burning. This means you start with the hardest exercise variation you can handle for a given movement for the first 30 seconds (such as Feet-Elevated Pushups) and then immediately drop to a slightly easier exercise variation for the final 30 seconds (like floor Pushups) to allow you to keep going. But that's getting ahead of ourselves. For starters, follow this structured program to a T and you'll reap incredible benefits, guaranteed.

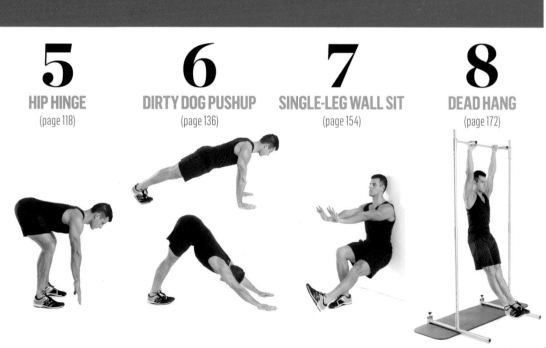

5 HIP HINGE (page 118)

6 DIRTY DOG PUSHUP (page 136)

7 SINGLE-LEG WALL SIT (page 154)

8 DEAD HANG (page 172)

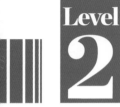

Beginner (28 Days)

1
SHOULDERS-ELEVATED HIP THRUST
(page 50)

2
PUSHUP
(page 68)

3
BOX SQUAT
(page 86)

4
ROW
(page 102)

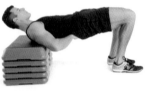
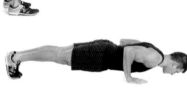
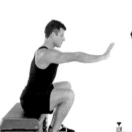
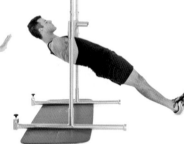

Level 3

Intermediate (28 Days)

1
FEET-ELEVATED HIP THRUST
(page 52)

2
SELF-ASSISTED SINGLE-ARM PUSHUP
(page 70)

3
DEEP SQUAT
(page 88)

4
SELF-ASSISTED SINGLE-ARM ROW
(page 104)

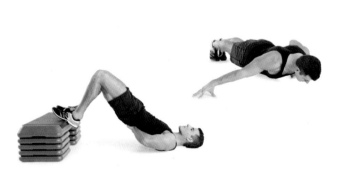
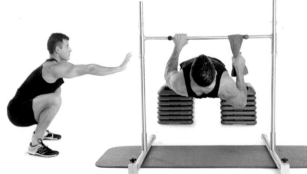

5
STAGGERED HIP HINGE
(page 120)

6
PUSH-AWAY
(page 138)

7
STEPUP
(page 156)

8
FLEXED HANG
(page 174)

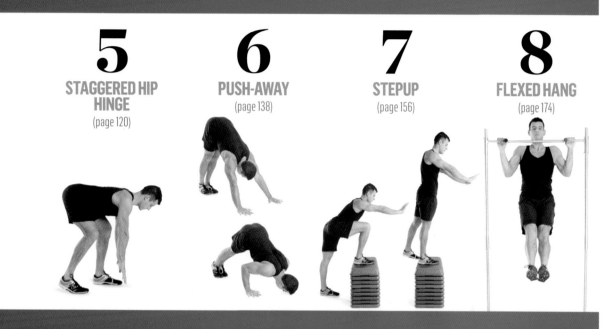

5
SINGLE-LEG HIP HINGE
(page 122)

6
PIKE PUSHUP
(page 140)

7
STAGGERED SQUAT
(page 158)

8
ECCENTRIC PULLUP
(page 176)

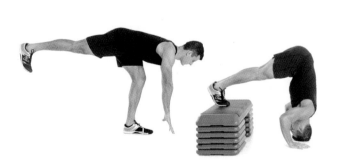

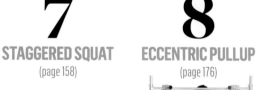
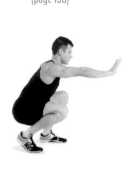
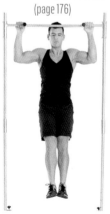
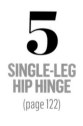

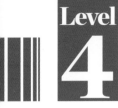

Level 4 — Advanced (28 Days)

1
SHOULDERS- AND FEET-ELEVATED HIP THRUST
(page 54)

2
SINGLE-ARM PUSHUP
(page 72)

3
DEEP OVERHEAD SQUAT
(page 90)

4
SINGLE-ARM ROW
(page 106)

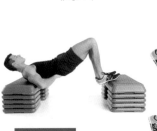

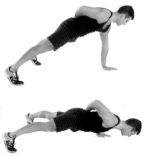

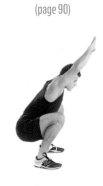

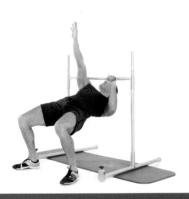

Level 5 — Superhero (28 Days)

1
SINGLE-LEG HIP THRUST
(page 56)

2
PLYOMETRIC PUSHUP
(page 74)

3
JUMP SQUAT
(page 92)

4
PLYOMETRIC ROW
(page 108)

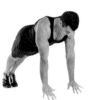

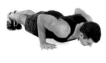

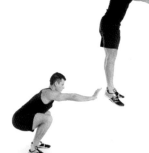

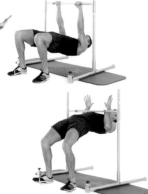

5
VERTICAL JUMP
(page 124)

6
HANDSTAND PUSHUP
(page 142)

7
LUNGE
(page 160)

8
PULLUP
(page 178)

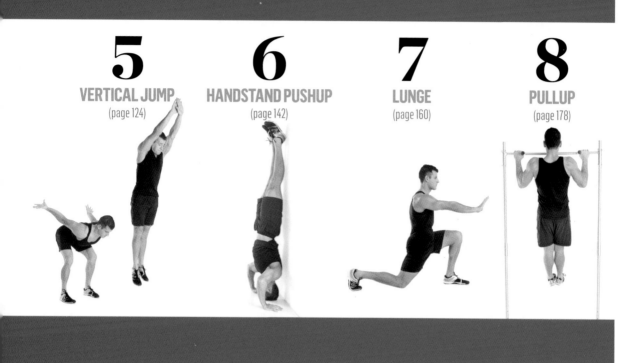

5
STAGGERED VERTICAL JUMP
(page 126)

6
SELF-ASSISTED SINGLE-ARM HANDSTAND PUSHUP
(page 144)

7
SINGLE-LEG SQUAT
(page 162)

8
SELF-ASSISTED SINGLE-ARM PULLUP
(page 180)

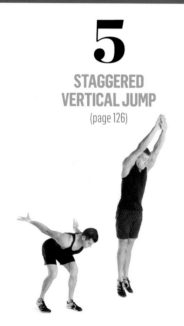
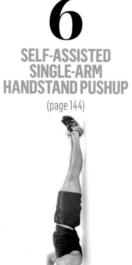
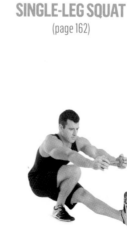
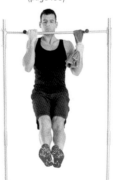
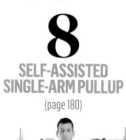

Chapter 14

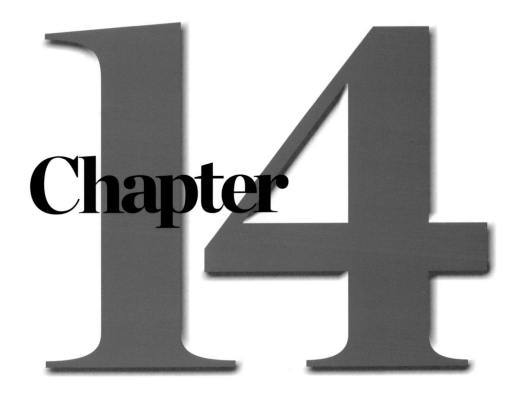

THE WORKOUTS

8 CHALLENGING ROUTINES FOR FAT-BURNING, STRENGTH, AND ENDURANCE!

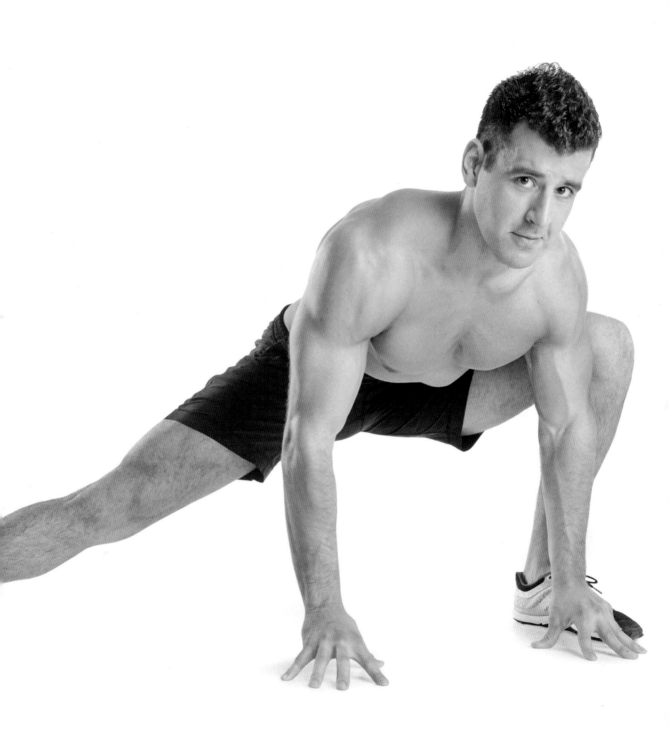

Everyone, it seems, wants to lose body fat. But there are a lot of other worthwhile motivations for fitness, and bodyweight training can help you achieve those, too.

In this chapter, you'll find workouts for just about every goal, whether you're looking for rapid fat loss, striving for serious muscle gain, or trying to build strength, power, or endurance. There are workouts for people with a minimalist approach to fitness or those looking to work their upper or lower body separately. If you find yourself really short on time, use the 8-minute workout to get your fat-burning on without needing to completely overhaul your busy schedule. There's something for everyone and every goal. Here are the workouts and how to build them into your life.

The BODYWEIGHT 8 W

1 2 3

BODYWEIGHT BUILDERS **THE MINIMALIST** **PURE POWER**

How many weeks do you perform each workout?

Well, the answer depends on your fitness level, goals, and training schedule. If all you care about is fat loss, you can keep rocking the Bodyweight Burners from Chapter 13 until the end of time as long as you switch up the exercise variations you're using every 2 to 4 weeks. If you want to regularly rotate between different training goals, you can jump to a new one of this chapter's workouts every 4 to 12 weeks. Beginners will do better by switching less frequently (every 6 to 12 weeks), where advanced trainees will do better shaking it up more often (every 2 to 4 weeks).

The most important thing to remember is the concept of progressive overload. This means you need to keep challenging your muscles with harder exercise variations to reach your goals.

kouts

4
SUPER STRENGTH

5
EXTREME ENDURANCE

6
THE 8-MINUTE WORKOUT

7
ULTIMATE UPPER- AND LOWER- BODY WORKOUTS

8
THE SHREDDER

No other exercise variable is more important than training intensity, which is why shorter 10- to 30-minute workouts can be so effective if you push yourself hard enough. That's why you spent so much time learning all of the exercise progressions. It's paramount that you continually reference the step-by-step progressions for the Bodyweight 8 exercises in Chapters 5 through 12 to completely customize your fitness experience for each workout. You'll be using the easier exercise variations for warmups and higher-rep endurance workouts and the harder exercises to build muscle and strength. Sometimes, you'll be using multiple exercise variations of varied levels of difficulty within the same training session. But don't sweat the details. It's easy to get caught in paralysis by analysis by trying to find your perfect workout program. Just pick a workout and get started right away. Remember: This chapter is for more flexible exercisers. If you prefer more variety, feel free to change between different workouts as much as you'd like. All that matters is that you train consistently, you work hard, and you make sure that you progress on a daily, weekly, and monthly basis by advancing to harder moves. If you find yourself in need of a rest week every once in a while, feel free to take one. Just be sure to still be active that week: Walk, play recreational sports, stretch, foam roll, and otherwise move around. Most people could do with an active recovery week every 6 to 12 weeks or so based on their training schedules, age, and fitness level.

#1
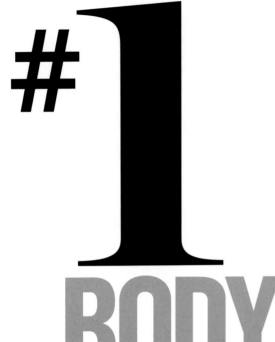

BODYWEIGHT BUILDERS

This simple and effective muscle-building program uses nothing but your body weight. Here we will alternate between an upper-body and a lower-body workout to allow your muscles more time for recovery (and growth) between workouts. Select the exercises that are right for your level of fitness. But keep in mind that you'll want to choose moves that are challenging enough

in the classic bodybuilding rep range of 6 to 12 reps instead of working for time as you do with workouts designed for fat loss. Since your legs are stronger than your arms, you may need to use single-leg exercises or add an external load like a weight vest, dumbbell, or kettlebell to the lower-body exercises.

Here's how it works

Perform four workouts per week, alternating between an upper-body workout and a lower-body workout. In each workout, alternate between two exercises that work opposing muscle groups; that's known as a superset format. You are free to choose the exercise level and variation you wish as long as you can complete the reps with good form. Complete a superset of 6 to 12 reps per exercise every 5 minutes. Perform 6 total supersets for a 30-minute workout. Your weekly training schedule is outlined below.

Use the first superset in each workout as a warmup. Choose easier exercise variations of the basic move for 10 to 20 reps to warm your muscles, lubricate your joints, and groove your movement patterns. Then perform the remaining 5 supersets in a rep range of 6 to 12.

For best results, you must perform your reps with a 3-2-1-1 training tempo to maximize time under tension. This means you'll take 3 seconds during the lowering portion, hold the finishing position for 2 seconds, take 1 second during the lifting portion, and then take 1 second to reset between each rep.

Once you can perform 5 sets of 12+ reps for a given exercise variation, you must move to the next level of progression in order to keep stimulating muscle growth.

If you're performing a unilateral exercise other than a Single-Leg Squat for Lower-Body Workout B, you'll need to perform 6 to 12 reps per side within each 5-minute superset block. For example, if you were performing a superset of Single-Arm Pushups and Single-Arm Rows, you would need to complete 6 to 12 reps per arm and leg for each move within a 5-minute time frame.

If you'd like, for the 6th and final superset, you can back off to an easier exercise variation and perform as many good reps as you can for a serious muscle pump. For example, if you were using Feet-Elevated Pushups for sets of 6 to 12 reps, back off to regular Push-ups for reps of 15 or more. You can perform these reps faster, still emphasizing a slower lowering speed.

If you find that you have a lot of extra rest time between sets, use exercise fillers like self-massage (foam rolling) or stretching/mobility work to fill in the gaps.

Exercise	Workout A		Workout B	
	MONDAY Upper Body	**TUESDAY** Lower Body	**THURSDAY** Upper Body	**FRIDAY** Lower Body
1	Pushup Variation	Deep Squat Variation	Handstand Pushup Variation	Single-Leg Squat Variation (Left Leg)
2	Row Variation	Hip Thrust or Hip Hinge Variation	Pullup Variation	Single-Leg Squat Variation (Right Leg)

#2

THE MINIMALIST

This workout is for someone who prefers a workout program that focuses on fewer movements and fewer total workouts per week.

It's a total-body workout in just three exercises. Do it once or twice a week. You'll still burn fat, build muscle, and boost metabolism, but you'll do it with the least effort possible.

Here's how it works

Alternate between the three exercises in the chart during each workout.

- If your goal is to build strength and power, perform as many sets of 3 to 5 reps for each exercise as you can in a 30-minute time frame. Only rest as much as needed between exercises, and be sure to choose exercise variations that challenge you in a 3- to 5-rep range.

- If your goal is to build muscle, perform as many sets of 6 to 12 reps for each exercise as you can in 30 minutes. Rest only as much as needed between exercises, and be sure to choose exercise variations that challenge you in a 6- to 12-rep range.

- If your goal is to build endurance, perform as many sets of 15 to 20 reps for each exercise as you can in 30 minutes. Only rest as much as needed between exercises, and be sure to choose exercise variations that challenge you in a 15- to 20-rep range.

- Use the first 1 or 2 sets for each exercise in each workout as a warmup by using an easier variation.

- If your goal is to train multiple muscle qualities within the same training session, then in every triset, mix between the various rep ranges mentioned above.

- Make certain you mix between the different exercise options within each Big Bodyweight 3 category from workout to workout (for example, mix between Pushups and Handstand Pushup variations).

- Be sure to perform an equal number of sets per side for all unilateral exercises, unless you are trying to strengthen an imbalance between sides by doing more total sets on the weak side.

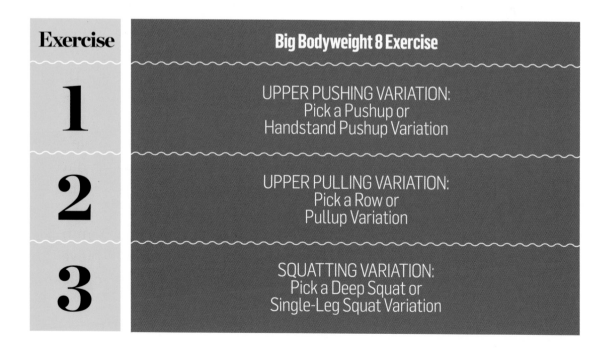

Exercise	Big Bodyweight 8 Exercise
1	UPPER PUSHING VARIATION: Pick a Pushup or Handstand Pushup Variation
2	UPPER PULLING VARIATION: Pick a Row or Pullup Variation
3	SQUATTING VARIATION: Pick a Deep Squat or Single-Leg Squat Variation

#3 PURE POWER

Power is moving your body as quickly as possible. To build it, use easier to moderately difficult bodyweight exercise variations. Power engages what's called the stretch reflex, or the rubber band–like qualities of your muscles and tendons. These explosive muscular contractions target your fast-twitch muscle fibers, which are key because they burn the most calories and have the largest impact on your metabolic rate. Power moves also elevate your heart rate higher than any other movement and enhance your athletic performance. In fact, circuiting a handful of bodyweight power training moves that work your whole body for only 20 minutes will have a ridiculous metabolic impact that rivals that of sprinting. A power workout is inherently higher impact, so it should be done only if you've been exercising regularly for at least 3 months.

Here's how it works

Perform this 20-minute total-body workout two or three times per week with ideally 48 hours between workouts. You could also alternate between this workout, Super Strength, and Extreme Endurance to train every key muscle quality within a given training week.

Alternate between 20 seconds of work and 40 seconds of rest for each exercise in the bodyweight circuit in the chart.

Completing the four exercises is one cycle. Perform up to five total cycles for a 20-minute workout.

Before you start the workout, perform 10 to 20 reps of an easier exercise variation for each move in the circuit to warm up your muscles, lubricate your joints, and groove your movement patterns.

If you prefer to work for reps instead of time, perform 5 to 10 reps of each exercise every minute and use the remainder of each minute to rest and transition to the next exercise.

For all unilateral exercises, switch sides at the halfway 10-second mark and perform an equal number of reps on each side. If you find that 10 seconds isn't enough time to get in enough work, perform 20 seconds on each side with no rest between sides. This will still give you 20 seconds of rest and transition time until you start the next exercise within the circuit. You could also perform 5 to 10 reps per side and use the remainder of that minute to rest.

These reps should be performed nearly continuously for maximum benefit and to get enough reps within each 20-second work period.

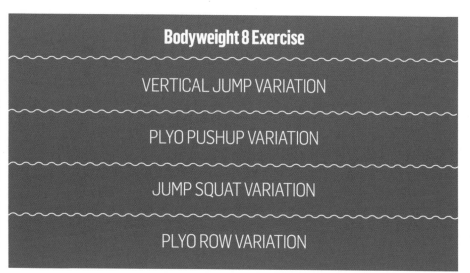

Exercise	Bodyweight 8 Exercise
1	VERTICAL JUMP VARIATION
2	PLYO PUSHUP VARIATION
3	JUMP SQUAT VARIATION
4	PLYO ROW VARIATION

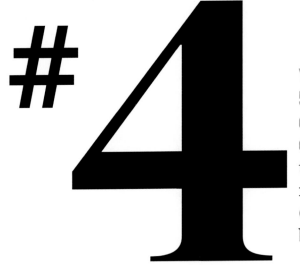

#4

You will develop maximal strength in a 3- to 5-rep range using heavy loads or advanced exercise variations performed at slower, more controlled tempos. The one drawback of traditional strength training is that it requires long and boring rest periods (often 3 to 5 minutes or longer) between sets, leaving many people

SUPER STRENGTH

feeling like they didn't sweat or work hard enough. So I've created a 20-minute strength circuit where you minimize workout time without sacrificing results. The cool thing about this setup is that you end up getting more than 4 minutes of rest before repeating the same exercise again while you're working other muscle groups. This keeps the intensity high for a serious calorie-burning and cardio boost.

Here's how it works

Perform this 20-minute total-body workout two or three times per week with ideally 48 hours between workouts. You could also alternate between this workout, Pure Power, and Extreme Endurance to train every key muscle quality within a given training week.

Alternate between 30 seconds of work and 30 seconds of rest for each exercise in the following bodyweight circuit.

Completing the five exercises is one cycle. Perform up to four total cycles for a 20-minute workout.

For best results, perform your reps with a 3-1-1-1 training tempo to maximize time under tension. This means you'll take 3 seconds during the lowering portion, hold the finishing position for 1 second, take 1 second during the lifting portion, and then take 1 second to reset between each rep. Over the course of 30 seconds, you could do at most 5 total reps.

Before you start the workout, perform 10 to 20 reps of an easier exercise variation for each move in the circuit to warm up.

If you prefer to work for reps instead of time, perform 3 to 5 reps of each exercise every minute and use the remainder of each minute to rest and transition to the next exercise.

For all unilateral exercises, switch sides at the halfway 15-second mark and perform an equal number of reps on each side. If you find that 15 seconds isn't enough time to get in enough work, stay on the same side the whole set and switch sides from cycle to cycle (making sure to perform an even number of total cycles, either two or four). You could also perform 3 to 5 reps per side and use the remainder of that minute to rest and transition to the next exercise.

Exercise	Bodyweight 8 Exercise
1	HIP THRUST VARIATION
2	PUSHUP OR HANDSTAND PUSHUP VARIATION
3	SINGLE-LEG SQUAT VARIATION (Left Side)
4	SINGLE-LEG SQUAT VARIATION (Right Side)
5	ROW OR PULLUP VARIATION

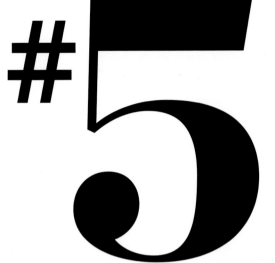

#5

This creates a surge of blood and nutrients to your muscles and builds up your lactic acid tolerance, or your ability to handle the burning sensation in your muscles that comes with higher-rep training. Your lower body has more natural muscular endurance

EXTREME ENDURANCE

than your upper body because it's used more often, so you'll find that upper-body moves are difficult to maintain for $1\frac{1}{2}$ minutes. Either employ short 3- to 5-second rest periods when needed or regress the exercise. Another option: Do a drop set. Perform the harder exercise variation for the first 45 seconds and then immediately regress to an easier move for the final 45 seconds.

Here's how it works

Perform this 20-minute total-body workout two or three times per week with ideally 48 hours between workouts. You could also alternate between this workout, Pure Power, and Super Strength to train every key muscle quality within a given training week.

Alternate between 1½ minutes of work and 30 seconds of rest for each exercise in the chart. Completing these five exercises is one cycle. Perform up to two total cycles for a 20-minute workout.

You can do these reps faster than you would with the Super Strength workout but still take a little longer during the lowering portion to relieve pressure on your joints and make your muscles work harder.

Before you start each workout, do 10 to 20 reps of an easier exercise variation for each move in the circuit to warm up your muscles, lubricate your joints, and groove your movement patterns.

If you prefer to work for reps instead of time, perform 15 to 20+ reps of each exercise every 2 minutes and use the remainder of each 2-minute block to rest and transition to the next exercise.

For all unilateral exercises, switch sides at the halfway 45-second mark and perform an equal number of reps on each side. If you find that 45 seconds isn't enough time to get in enough work, stay on the same side the whole set and switch sides from cycle to cycle. You could also perform 15 to 20 reps per side and use the remainder of that 2-minute block to rest and transition to the next exercise.

Exercise	Bodyweight 8 Exercise
1	HIP THRUST VARIATION
2	PUSHUP OR HANDSTAND PUSHUP VARIATION
3	SINGLE-LEG SQUAT VARIATION (Left Side)
4	SINGLE-LEG SQUAT VARIATION (Right Side)
5	ROW OR PULLUP VARIATION

#6

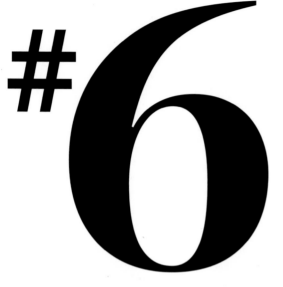

THE 8-MINUTE WORKOUT

While most people can find 30 to 60 minutes to train a couple times per week, there will be days where things get so busy you'll only have 10 minutes to spare. Well, 10 minutes is way better than nothing! In fact, a recent study showed that a 10-minute workout had the same postworkout metabolic boost as a 30-minute workout, though the 30-minute workout burned more total calories during the session due to the higher exercise volume. The key with a shorter workout is intensity. With such a low total exercise volume, you really have to push yourself outside of your comfort zone and take little to no rest between exercises in order to get a good workout.

Here's how it works

Alternate between 50 seconds of hard work and 10 seconds of rest for each exercise in the following bodyweight circuit.

Perform as many reps as you can with perfect form within each 50-second work period. If it's an isometric exercise, simply hold the position for as long as you can. If you need to rest or pause at any point, please do so. Your goal is to eventually be able to continuously work for the full 50 seconds without stopping.

For all unilateral exercises, be sure to switch sides at the halfway mark so you perform 25 seconds of work on each side.

You should be able to perform at least 10 total reps (5 per side for a unilateral movement) within each 50-second work period. If you're consistently getting fewer than 10 total reps, make the exercise easier by using one of the microregressions within each exercise level. If you're consistently getting more than 10 total reps, make the exercise harder by using one of the microprogressions within each exercise level. You can also feel free to mix and match between other variations of a given exercise level, if you'd like.

If you're using plyometric exercises like Jump Squats or Plyo Rows, pause for 4 to 5 seconds in the top or bottom position between explosive reps to emphasize quality over quantity. You can also alternate between 10 seconds of work and 10 seconds of rest three times to fill the full minute.

Exercise	Bodyweight 8 Exercise
1	HIP THRUST VARIATION
2	PUSHUP VARIATION
3	DEEP SQUAT VARIATION
4	ROW VARIATION
5	HIP HINGE VARIATION
6	HANDSTAND PUSHUP VARIATION
7	SINGLE-LEG SQUAT VARIATION
8	PULLUP VARIATION

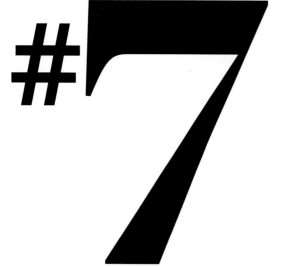

#7

These workouts are inspired by German Volume Training (GVT), a program in which you do 10 sets of 10 reps of an exercise for a certain movement pattern or muscle group. I've modified them to use more functional bodyweight exercises that work multiple muscle groups at once so you don't have to train one body part per day.

ULTIMATE UPPER- AND LOWER-BODY WORKOUTS

Here's how the Upper-Body Workout works

Perform two upper-body workouts per week, taking at least 72 hours of rest in between. Each workout consists of a superset of a pushing exercise and pulling exercise.

In Workout A, alternate between a Pushup and Row variation that you are strong enough to do for 12 to 15 reps in a single set.

In Workout B, alternate between a Handstand Pushup and Pullup variation that you are strong enough to do for 12 to 15 reps in a single set.

Try to perform 10 reps of each exercise within the superset every 4 minutes. Do 10 total supersets for a 40-minute workout.

You most likely will not be able to perform 10 reps for all 10 sets; bump down to 9, 8, 7, 6, or even 5 reps toward the last sets. Once you can do 10 reps for all 10 sets, advance to a harder variation.

Before you start each workout, perform 10 to 20 reps of an easier exercise variation for each move in the superset to warm up.

For the unilateral exercises, you may need to perform 5 reps per side to get your 10 total reps.

Here's how the Lower-Body Workout works

Perform two lower-body workouts per week taking at least 72 hours of rest in between. Each workout consists of a superset of a single-leg exercise.

In Workout A, alternate between right and left sides of a Single-Leg Squat variation that you are strong enough to do for 12 to 15 reps per side.

In Workout B, alternate between right and left sides of a Single-Leg Hip Thrust or Hip Hinge variation that you can do for 12 to 15 reps per side.

Try to perform 10 reps on each side every 4 minutes. Do 10 total supersets for a 40-minute workout.

You most likely will not be able to perform 10 reps for all 10 sets; bump down to 9, 8, 7, 6, or even 5 reps toward the last sets. Once you can do 10 reps for all 10 sets, advance to a harder variation.

Before you start each workout, perform 10 to 20 reps of an easier exercise variation for each move in the superset to warm up.

	Workout A		Workout B	
Exercise	**MONDAY** Upper Body	**TUESDAY** Lower Body	**THURSDAY** Upper Body	**FRIDAY** Lower Body
1	PUSHUP VARIATION	SINGLE-LEG SQUAT VARIATION	HANDSTAND PUSHUP VARIATION	SINGLE-LEG HIP THRUST OR HINGE VARIATION
2	ROW VARIATION	SINGLE-LEG SQUAT VARIATION (Other Leg)	PULLUP VARIATION	SINGLE-LEG HIP THRUST OR HINGE VARIATION (Other Leg)

#8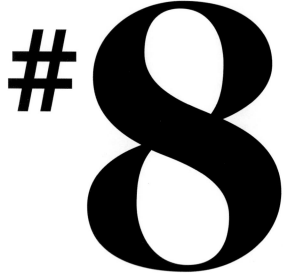

This is my go-to routine when I'm trying to get really lean for a photo shoot. To torch fat and still maintain muscle mass, I start with a 40-minute strength-training circuit that works my whole body using harder exercises, lower reps, and longer rest periods. Then I finish with 20 minutes of a

THE SHREDDER

classic metabolic-resistance-training (MRT) circuit. This provides the best of both exercise styles. If you want to focus more on fat loss, bump up the MRT circuit to 30 minutes and bump down the strength work to 30 minutes. Just keep the total workout to 60 minutes or fewer.

Here's how it works

Perform this whole-body workout three times per week with ideally 48 hours between workouts.

This workout has two parts to be performed in this order:

Part I—Heavy strength-training circuit: 40 minutes

Part II—Metabolic-resistance-training circuit: 20 minutes

FOR PART I, perform one cycle within 10 minutes. Take ample rest between each exercise to keep intensity high, and use any remaining time to do active recovery like foam rolling or stretching.

"Heavy" means you select a variation of each exercise that challenges you in a 3- to 6-rep range using the Bodyweight 8 exercise progressions. For all unilateral exercises, be sure to perform 3 to 6 reps on each side within each 10-minute time frame.

Perform four cycles for 40 total minutes. Use easier exercise variations in the first cycle to warm up.

FOR PART II, perform 60 seconds of work and 15 seconds of rest for each exercise in the chart.

That's one cycle. Perform four total cycles for about 20 total minutes and then grab a cold shower!

Use variations of these exercises that are significantly easier than the ones you used for the heavy strength work so you can get 10 reps to 20 reps within every 60-second work period.

For all unilateral exercises, be sure to switch sides at the halfway mark so you perform 30 seconds of work on each side. You could also perform all your reps or work on one side and then switch sides from cycle to cycle, if you'd like. Just make sure to perform an equal number of reps on each side and perform an even number of total sets.

Part I
Heavy Strength-Training Circuit
HEAVY SQUATTING EXERCISE
HEAVY PULLING EXERCISE
HEAVY PUSHING EXERCISE

Part II
Metabolic-Resistance-Training Circuit
HIP THRUST OR HIP HINGE VARIATION
PUSHUP OR HANDSTAND PUSHUP VARIATION
DEEP SQUAT OR SINGLE-LEG SQUAT VARIATION
ROW OR PULLUP VARIATION

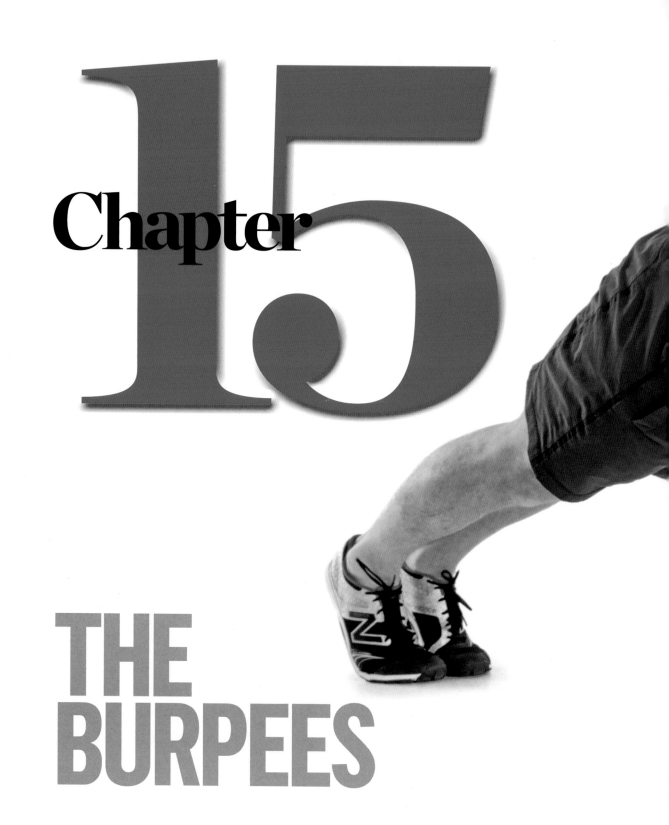

Chapter 15

THE BURPEES

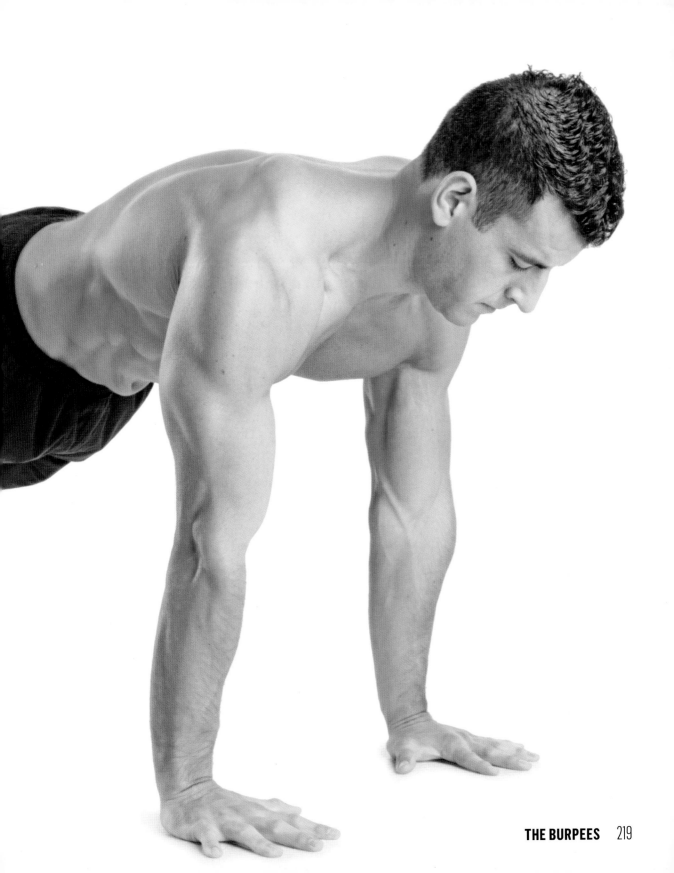

You are probably familiar with interval training, the holy grail of fat-loss workouts. In interval training, you alternate between periods of intense work and active recovery. There is a ton of research to show how effective interval training is for fat loss and improving fitness. A recent study in the *Journal of Physiology* found that interval training at a high intensity on a bike can provide all the health and fitness benefits of riding continuously but more slowly for a far longer period of time. Short bursts working at 75 percent of your maximum heart rate or higher will boost your metabolism, burn more fat at rest, and earn you the muscular physique of a sprinter rather than the slight frame of an endurance athlete. Another bonus: Interval-training sessions

can be completed in 20 to 30 minutes or fewer, and all it takes is several weekly sessions to get great results—making this training style the ideal solution for busy people needing to burn belly fat.

Whether or not you are pressed for time, you should incorporate interval training (also called metabolic training) into your fitness program. In the next chapter, you'll learn my eight favorite bodyweight cardio moves that I believe will soon become your favorites, too. But first, let's take a long look at the biggest, baddest cardio-interval-metabolic exercise of all time. If I were imprisoned on a desert island and my evil captors locked me in a cage only about the length of my body, I could still stay in fighting shape by doing only one exercise in that limited space—the Burpee.

The Burpee is the baddest bodyweight exercise in existence, an incredible whole-body muscle builder, fat burner, and metabolism booster that will also make you more athletic for sport. Pure and simple, Burpees suck! If you've done them, you know what I mean. A workout of Burpees is like going several rounds with Mike Tyson in his prime. When my boot

campers or clients hear that Burpees are on the agenda for a workout, they take a deep breath, a heavy gulp, and pray to the fitness gods for courage to get through the hellfire coming their way.

The Burpee movement can be traced to the work of American physiologist Royal H. Burpee in the 1930s. He developed the move as a quick and easy test to assess total-body fitness. The exercise continued to gain popularity through use in military boot camps and, later, as the calisthenic cardio exercise of choice in gym classes and athletic practices worldwide.

This ultimate equipment-free total-body exercise consists of a series of smooth and fluid movements that take your body from full standing to a Pushup position and back. It combines hip hinging, squatting, planking, pushing, and jumping movements into one seamless sweat maker. No other exercise works more muscles and burns more calories per minute than the big nasty Burpee. Perfect execution of this move is also a sign of elite athleticism and functional fitness. Did I mention that they suck?

The Burpee is a whole-body up-and-down metabolic nightmare. And it's complicated to perform, which is why it is often bastardized by those who attempt it without proper instruction. It's fraught with problems. But I'm about to show you how to properly perform the Burpee and make some instant modifications that will immediately boost performance and reduce the risk of injury. Plus, I provide you with a five-step exercise progression system that will have you going beast mode with Burpees in no time! The result will be a more refined Burpee routine that very well may break your heart, mind, and soul but not your body. That we'll leave to Mr. Tyson.

HOW TO PERFORM THE PERFECT BURPEE

Stand with your feet hip-width apart. Squat down low enough so that your hands touch the floor without rounding your lower back and while keeping your feet flat. Kick your legs back into a Pushup position with your back flat and then quickly return to the squatting position. Stand and repeat. That's 1 rep of a Burpee. You can also add a full-range-of-motion Pushup while in the Pushup position and add a jump when standing up from the Deep Squat position. Now before you go nuts with this, start out slowly and get the movement down. There are several ways to instantly improve your Burpee performance.

❶ Perform it through a modified range of motion with your hands placed on a stable low box, step, couch, or ottoman. This move, the Low-Box Burpee, is the ground zero exercise in my Burpee progression.

❷ Use a wider stance with your feet shoulder-width apart or slightly wider. This makes it easier to get your hands on the floor because it doesn't require as much range of motion at the hips. In turn, this makes it easier to keep your back flat so you don't look like a crouching fool in the bottom position.

❸ Really slow down the movement and break it up into its component parts. On the next two pages, you'll learn how to do a special Burpee mobility test that isolates each move and determines if you are flexible enough to do Burpees without risk of injury. This movement screen is called the Blocked-Feet Burpee Mobility Test. By "blocked feet" I mean feet together. You should keep your feet together throughout the assessment.

Blocking your feet together makes the movement harder, but it forces you to learn good squatting and jumping mechanics because it makes you keep your feet flat, toes forward, and knees out. One of the scariest things I've seen with Burpees is how much the knees can collapse inward during the squatting or landing portions of the exercise, opening up the exercise to the risk of an ACL tear. With your feet together, the farthest your knees can drive inward is until they touch, which is still a safe position.

Because blocked feet force you through a greater range of motion, you naturally must slow down the movement, which is safer. In addition, it makes it easier for you to engage your core, because you can squeeze your legs together and clench your glutes better. This is particularly important for protecting your lower back when transitioning in and out of the Pushup position.

When performing the Blocked-Feet Burpee test, be sure to use the proper Hip-Hinge technique you learned in Chapter 6. Do each step in the movement on the next page slowly as if each were a separate rep. Practice your form and evaluate your mobility. Master this and you will be ready for the feet-apart Burpee and its many fat-torching iterations.

Blocked-Feet Burpee Mobility Test

YOU CAN USE THIS TEST AS A WARMUP OR ACTIVE RECOVERY BETWEEN WORKOUTS.

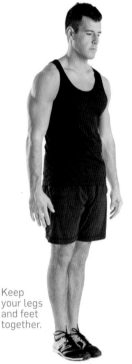

Keep your legs and feet together.

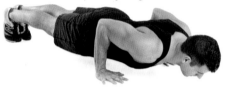

Perform a full Pushup (optional).

Squeeze your glutes.

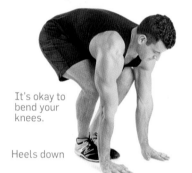

Minimize movement of your lower back.

It's okay to bend your knees.

Heels down

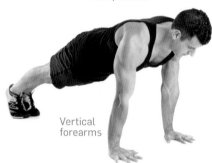

Plank position

Vertical forearms

1. THE START: Assume a standing hollow-body position with your feet placed together in tripod foot position. If you start in a strong and stable position, you have a better chance of finishing in a strong and stable position.

2. PLACE YOUR HANDS ON THE FLOOR: Push your knees out and perform a Hip Hinge, placing your palms flat on the floor directly underneath your shoulders. If you can't get your palms flat on the floor without rounding your back, it means that you're missing motion at your hips and hamstrings and you're better suited to performing a Low-Box Burpee.

3. JUMP YOUR FEET BACK INTO A PLANK: Depending on your fitness level, you can either hold this top Pushup (or Plank) position or perform a full-range-of-motion Pushup, keeping your forearms perpendicular to the floor throughout. A Low-Box Burpee allows you to perform an easier Hands-Elevated Pushup.

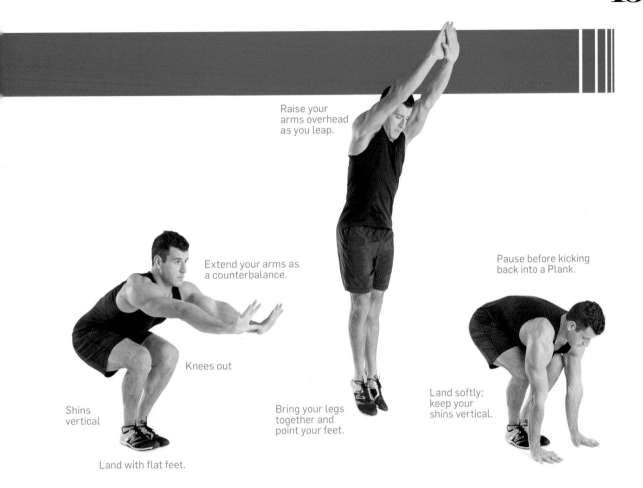

Raise your arms overhead as you leap.

Extend your arms as a counterbalance.

Knees out

Shins vertical

Land with flat feet.

Bring your legs together and point your feet.

Pause before kicking back into a Plank.

Land softly; keep your shins vertical.

4. JUMP YOUR FEET FORWARD INTO A SQUAT: Still keeping your feet together, drive your hips forward, pull your knees to your chest, and try to replace your hands with your feet so that your feet land right underneath your hips. You should land into the bottom of a Squat with your back flat, knees out, feet flat on the floor, and your arms fully extended in front of your body for counterbalance.

5. JUMP UPWARD: From the Squat position, forcefully extend your ankles, knees, and hips and reach your arms overhead. While airborne, you should assume a hollow-body position with your feet and legs together, armpits forward, and toes pointing down. This will provide you with the most core and shoulder stability midair.

6. LAND INTO THE NEXT REP: As the balls of your feet touch the ground with your feet still together, immediately bend your knees, drop your feet flat, and push your hips back. Your trunk will bend forward for counterbalance, which is fine as long as you keep your back flat. Land as softly as possible, with your shins perpendicular to the floor to protect your knees.

How did you do? If you struggled with any one of (or all of) the individual components—Hip Hinge, Squat, Pushup, jumping and landing—then you aren't ready for Burpees. Go back and practice the components separately and in combo until you can pass the test.

Yeah . . . the Burpee is complicated. That's because it's a bodyweight combination movement, which requires the greatest degree of total-body coordination and control. Once you can pass the Blocked-Feet Burpee

Mobility Test, use it as a warmup or for active recovery work between workouts. For best results, I would perform a couple sets of 5 to 10 reps every day. It's a corrective exercise that will make all other Burpees way easier to

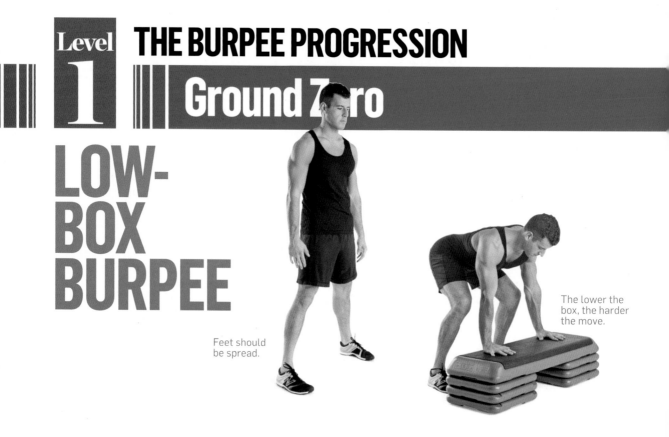

Level 1

THE BURPEE PROGRESSION
Ground Zero

LOW-BOX BURPEE

Feet should be spread.

The lower the box, the harder the move.

perform. Just be sure to do it super slow and with intention, holding and feeling every key position, so it takes about 10 seconds or so to perform each rep. If you really struggle with it, use the low-box setup and wide foot placement. It also never hurts to start with slower tempos and gradually build to faster tempos as you get deeper into your workout. From there, follow the Levels 1 through 5 progressions below.

Though not everyone can do Levels 3 to 5 on the floor, almost everyone can do them with a low-box setup that's elevated to knee height or higher. Always remember to take control of your workout and regress your Burpees as much as needed. Note that for the unilateral Burpee variations seen in Levels 3 through 5, you can perform all of your reps on one side and then switch sides from set to set, switch sides at the halfway mark of a given time-based work period, or alternate between sides every rep within the same work set.

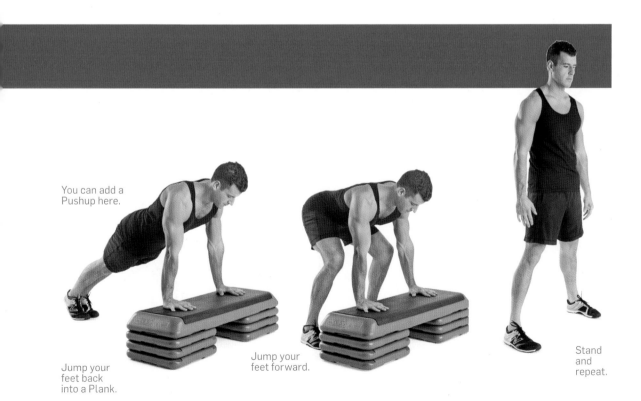

You can add a Pushup here.

Jump your feet back into a Plank.

Jump your feet forward.

Stand and repeat.

Level 2

Beginner

BURPEE

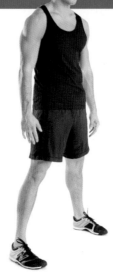

Perform a Hinging Squat.

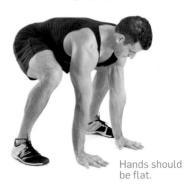

Hands should be flat.

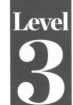

Level 3

Intermediate

SINGLE-LEG BURPEE

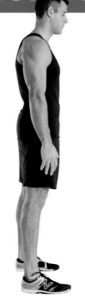

Upper back will round slightly.

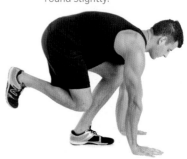

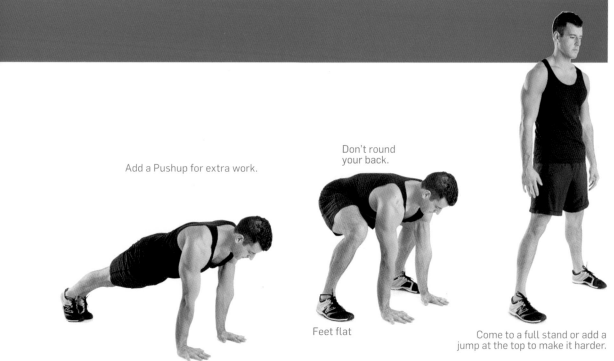

Add a Pushup for extra work.

Don't round your back.

Feet flat

Come to a full stand or add a jump at the top to make it harder.

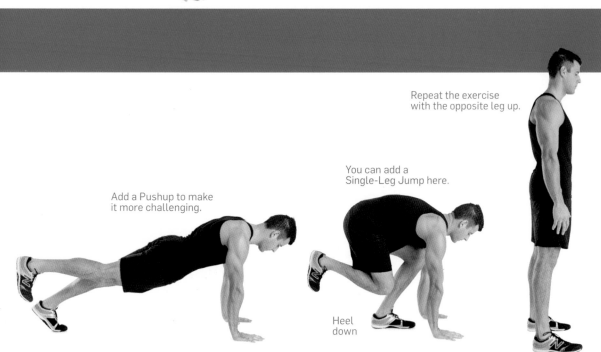

Repeat the exercise with the opposite leg up.

You can add a Single-Leg Jump here.

Add a Pushup to make it more challenging.

Heel down

4

Advanced

SINGLE-ARM BURPEE

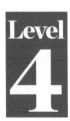

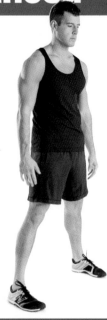

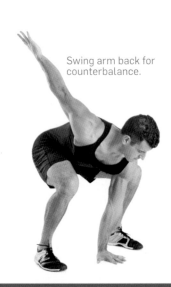

Swing arm back for counterbalance.

5

Superhero

SINGLE-ARM, SINGLE-LEG BURPEE

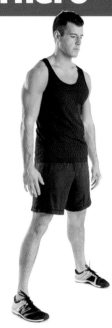

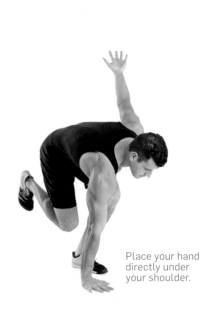

Place your hand directly under your shoulder.

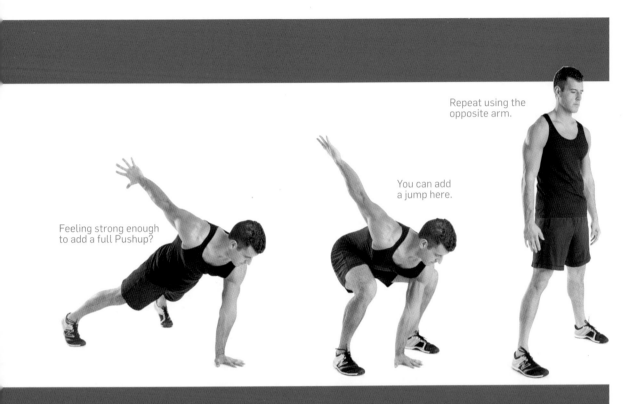

Feeling strong enough to add a full Pushup?

You can add a jump here.

Repeat using the opposite arm.

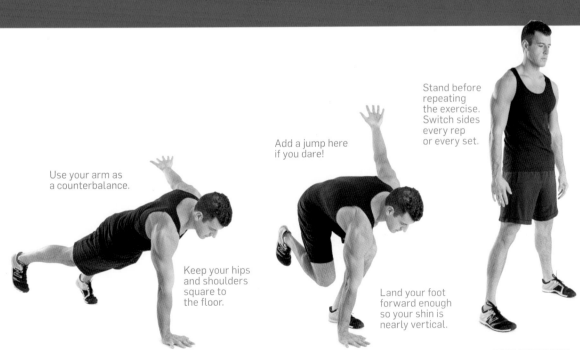

Use your arm as a counterbalance.

Keep your hips and shoulders square to the floor.

Add a jump here if you dare!

Land your foot forward enough so your shin is nearly vertical.

Stand before repeating the exercise. Switch sides every rep or every set.

THE BACKWARD BURPEE

The Backward Burpee is the opposite of the classic Burpee, which means it's done supine (facing up) instead of facing the floor. From a standing position, you perform a Deep Squat and sit down on the floor, then do a Backward Roll while keeping your abs crunched and braced and swinging your legs above you. Now, roll forward to move from a lying to a standing position without touching the floor with your hands or arms (you will, however, swing your arms forward for momentum). This makes the Backward Burpee more lower-body intensive

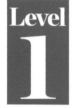

Level 1 | THE BACKWARD BURPEE PROGRESSION

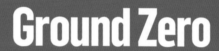

Ground Zero

FLEXED ROLL

Crunch your abs throughout the exercise.

Sit and roll back.

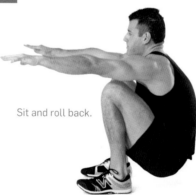
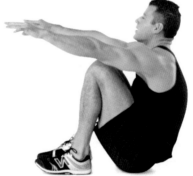

than a regular Burpee. Eventually, you're going to do this on only one leg at a time for an amazing body fat burner.

Outlined below and on the following pages is a complete step-by-step exercise progression sequence to take you from ground zero to superhero. You start learning how to safely roll on your back and progress to moving from a Roll to a Squat to standing and back. From there, you gradually build up the strength, balance, stability, and mobility to be able to roll from your back to a Single-Leg Squat to standing and back. In fact, Rolling Squats and Rolling Pistol Squats are great stepping-stone exercises to prepare you for

the demands of Deep Squats and Pistol Squats. The added momentum you generate with your arms and legs as you roll backward and forward makes it easier to stand up from a Deep Squat position, especially on one leg. Really focus on reaching your arms as far in front of your body as you can when rolling forward. Your trunk will bend forward, which is fine as long as you keep your back flat. You also have to get your feet directly underneath your hips as you transition to the Deep Squat position or you'll tip back a bit. Kick any of the Rolling Squat variations into overdrive by adding a jump at the top of the movement.

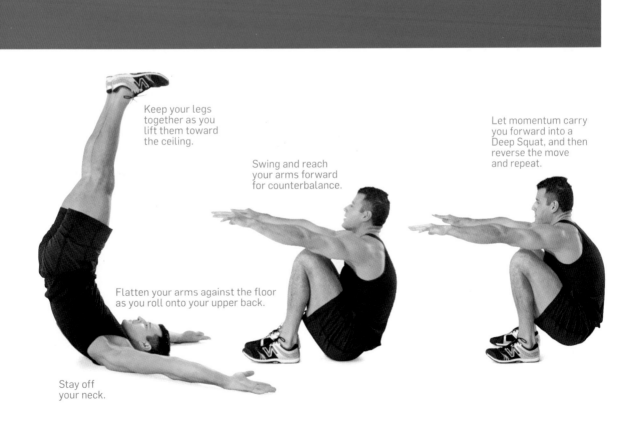

Keep your legs together as you lift them toward the ceiling.

Swing and reach your arms forward for counterbalance.

Let momentum carry you forward into a Deep Squat, and then reverse the move and repeat.

Flatten your arms against the floor as you roll onto your upper back.

Stay off your neck.

ROLLING SQUAT

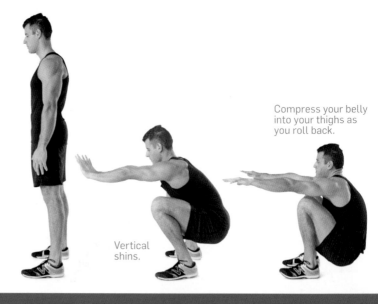

Compress your belly into your thighs as you roll back.

Vertical shins.

2 LEGS DOWN, 1 LEG UP

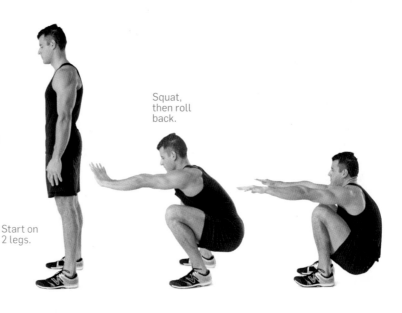

Squat, then roll back.

Start on 2 legs.

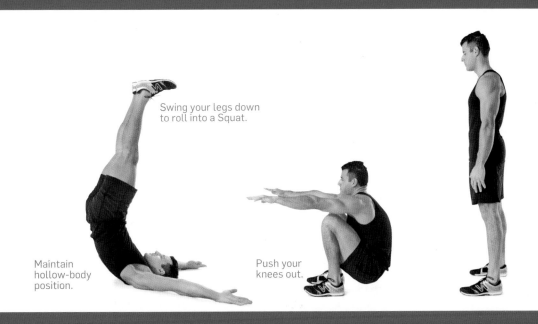

Swing your legs down to roll into a Squat.

Maintain hollow-body position.

Push your knees out.

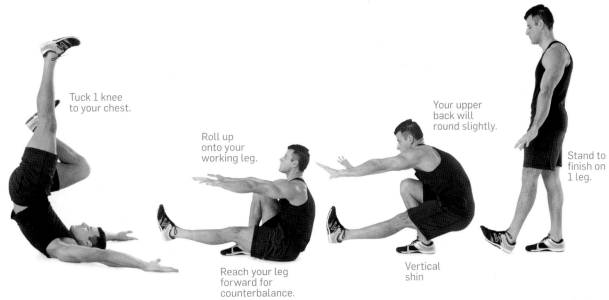

Tuck 1 knee to your chest.

Roll up onto your working leg.

Your upper back will round slightly.

Stand to finish on 1 leg.

Reach your leg forward for counterbalance.

Vertical shin

THE BURPEES 233

1 LEG DOWN, 2 LEGS' UP

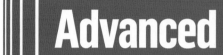

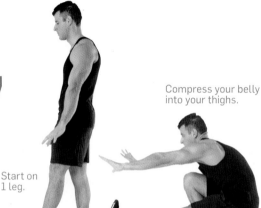

Start on 1 leg.

Elevate your leg.

Compress your belly into your thighs.

Roll back, keeping your core braced.

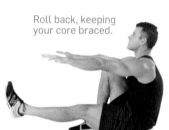

SINGLE-LEG BACKWARD BURPEE OR ROLLING PISTOL SQUAT

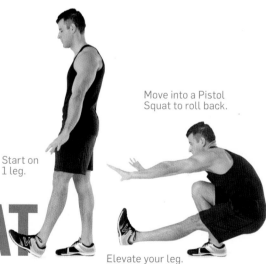

Start on 1 leg.

Elevate your leg.

Move into a Pistol Squat to roll back.

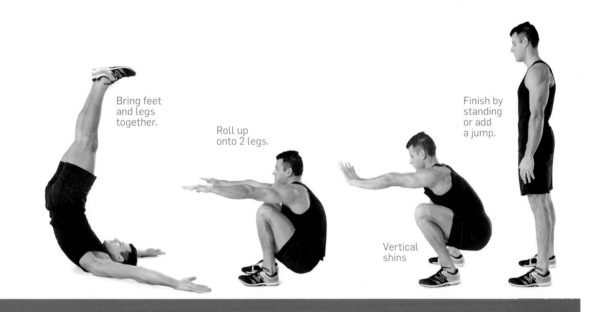

Bring feet
and legs
together.

Roll up
onto 2 legs.

Finish by
standing
or add
a jump.

Vertical
shins

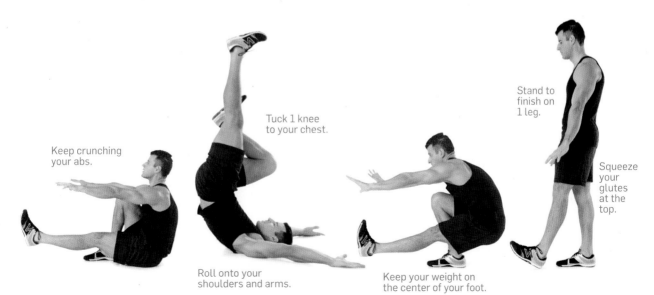

Keep crunching
your abs.

Tuck 1 knee
to your chest.

Stand to
finish on
1 leg.

Squeeze
your
glutes
at the
top.

Roll onto your
shoulders and arms.

Keep your weight on
the center of your foot.

Rolling on your thoracic through lumbar spine, or your upper through lower back using Backward Burpees, is a great way to make your spine more supple. The key thing to focus on is maintaining a hollow-body position and keeping your abs fully crunched and flexed as you roll one vertebra at a time. Where you can get into trouble is if you lose the braced core position and let your lower back hyperextend when you make contact with the ground. Avoid rolling onto your head and neck, which often happens when you let your legs come too far back behind your body instead of straight up to the sky as they should. I prefer to reach my arms overhead to make ground contact as I roll back because it allows me to prevent too much weight from shifting toward my neck. Going very slowly in the beginning, especially when rolling back, will clean up your technique. Finally, be sure to use a softer surface to roll onto like carpet, grass, or a padded mat to make the exercise a bit more comfortable.

If you find it too difficult to perform this move from the floor, modify it in a similar way as you did with the Burpee by using a low box setup. Basically, you perform a Rolling Box Squat where you rock your body back and lift your feet off the floor after moving into the seated position on the box, all while keeping your abs braced and flexed. Then you rock forward and quickly put your feet back on the ground and directly underneath your hips to stand right back up and repeat. You can, of course, progress to doing this on one leg at a time or adding a jump to the top of the movement.

THE SUPER BURPEE

If you're looking for one move that's guaranteed to put an "S" on your chest, it's this grotesque gut-buster. The Super Burpee combines a regular Burpee with a Backward Burpee for the best of both Burpee worlds.

Here are a handful of my favorite Super Burpee variations.

- Burpee and Backward Burpee (jump at the top of both movements)

- Single-Leg Burpee and Single-Leg Backward Burpee

- Single-Arm Burpee and Single-Leg Backward Burpee

THE WORKOUT FROM HELL

One of the bonus workouts in the Men's Health DeltaFit Speed Shred DVD series is called "The Workout from Hell" and features 60 minutes of nothing but Burpees. You alternate between 60 seconds of work and 60 seconds of rest for 30 total rounds, starting with the easiest Burpees in the beginning (Level 1) and progressing to harder Burpees from round to round, but only if you're ready for them. I've received tweets and Facebook messages from people around the world saying that this was the most challenging and most rewarding workout they've ever done. If 60 minutes is too long, just cut down the number of rounds as needed to completely customize your workout. Even five rounds will give you a great bodyweight cardio workout, and it only takes 10 minutes!

- Skater Jump Super Burpee (perform a Skater Jump [page 244] on each side at the transition between a Burpee and Backward Burpee)

- Mountain Climber Burpee (perform 3 to 5 seconds of Mountain Climbers [page 250] when in the Pushup position of a regular Burpee)

OTHER BURPEE VARIATIONS

To make Burpees more challenging, add other bodyweight cardio exercises at various points during the exercise. The following movements can be added when in the standing position.

- Jumping Jacks

- Skater Jumps

- Running or shuffling in place

- Any standing lower-body exercise (Squats, Lunges, Hip Hinges, Stepups, etc.)

- Punching or kicking

- Jumping Pullups

The following movements are appropriate to add when in the Pushup or Plank position.

- Mountain Climbers

- T-Pushups

- Plyometric Pushup variations

- Pushup to Plank Transfers

- Break-Dancers

- Donkey Kicks and other ground-based animal movements

The options are endless when it comes to Burpees, so keep an open mind, have fun, and be creative! If you're unfamiliar with any of these add-ons, many of them will be explained in the Bodyweight 8 Cardio exercises in the next chapter.

MY FAVORITE BURPEE WORKOUT

The one knock I'll give to the Burpee is that it doesn't work your upper-body pulling muscles. There are a couple ways you can remedy this. One, stand underneath a pullup bar and perform a Jumping Pullup while coming out of the Deep Squat position. Two, Dead Hang from a pullup bar and/or perform Pullups as active recovery between sets of Burpees. My favorite Burpee workout is where I set the clock for 10 minutes and do as many quality Burpees as I can. I stop whenever I need to catch my breath or I feel like I'm about to sacrifice form and technique. But instead of resting and doing nothing, I jump up on a pullup bar and do as many good Pullups as possible. When I can't do any more Pullups, I hang from the bar in a hollow-body position. When I'm ready to do Burpees again, I jump down and get back to work. Repeat this process until the time is up.

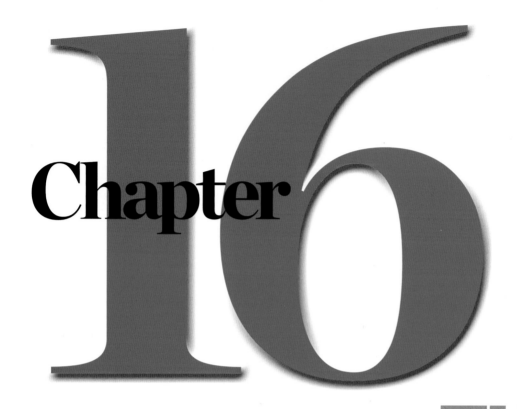

Chapter 16

THE BODYWEIGHT 8 CARDIO EXERCISES

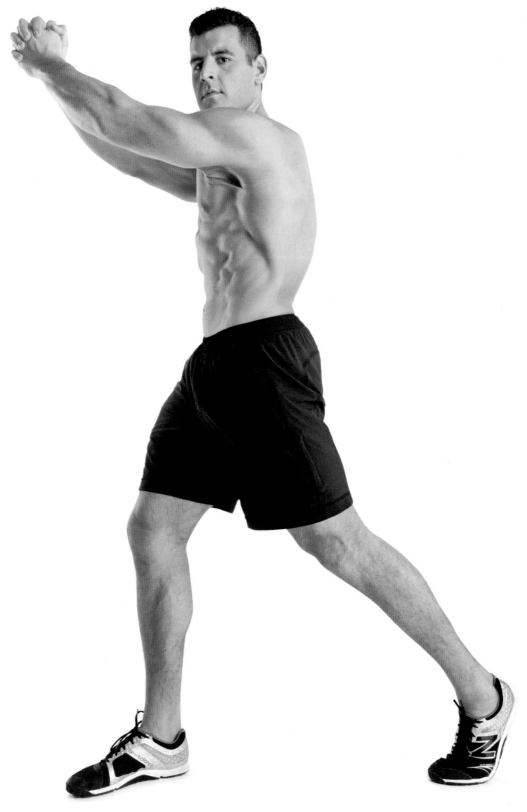

Metabolic training (MT) is the ultimate fusion of anaerobic strength training and aerobic cardio exercise. It's the best style of training to get you shredded as fast as possible.

The goal of this kind of workout is to create a massive metabolic disturbance to cause what's known as excess postexercise oxygen consumption, or EPOC, which reflects an elevated metabolic rate that lasts for up to 48 hours after completing your workout. This way, you're burning a bunch of calories both during your workout and long afterward during the recovery process. It's important to note that this "afterburn" phenomenon does not occur with typical aerobic exercise, such as a long, slow, 45-minute jog around the park. To enjoy the afterburn benefit, your workout needs *intensity* (you need to work very hard) and *density* (you need to accomplish a lot of "work" in a given period of time).

There are two main types of metabolic training to use to cause the fat-burning full-body disturbance that triggers EPOC.

1. **METABOLIC RESISTANCE TRAINING (MRT):** This is a muscle-and-strength style of interval training. Select several resistance-training exercises that work your entire body and then alternate between those moves with little to no rest. Work periods are typically 30 to 60 seconds at a time, and rest periods are typically 30 seconds or fewer. The Bodyweight Burners workouts in Chapter 13 are good examples. They allow you to simultaneously burn fat and build muscle.

2. **CARDIO INTERVAL TRAINING (CIT):** This is often referred to as high-intensity interval training (HIIT) and is classically performed by running outdoors or on a treadmill or by using a cardio machine like the recumbent bike or elliptical. An example of an HIIT running workout would be alternating between, say, 30 seconds of all-out sprinting and 1 minute of recovery while running at a moderate pace. For our purposes in this book, we'll be using bodyweight cardio exercises instead of running or spinning. One option is to select a single bodyweight cardio exercise that works your whole body, like a Burpee, and alternate between periods of intense work and active recovery. You can also select two or more noncompetitive bodyweight cardio exercises, like Jumping Jacks and Mountain Climbers, and alternate between them from set to set to keep intensity high.

In this chapter, we'll focus on the best cardio exercises you can do without equipment. There are eight of them, divided into two categories: four that primarily work your lower body and four that primarily work your upper body. I've grouped them for several reasons. One, this allows you to alternate between the upper- and lower-body cardio moves to keep intensity high, provide more exercise variety, and manage fatigue. Two, if you had a lower-body injury, you could use more of the upper-body cardio exercises, and vice versa. Three, most cardio exercises are skewed to work your legs instead of your arms. This leads to overuse injuries for the lower body and poor endurance for the upper body.

THE FOUR LOWER-BODY-INTENSIVE CARDIO MOVES

1. Jumping Jack
2. Skater Jump
3. Skier Swing
4. Sprinter

These are my selections, but keep in mind that you can use just about any Squat, Lunge, or Stepup variation that you can perform quickly to fit within the lower-body-intensive cardio category. Jump Squat variations also fit well if you're ready for them. I would still urge you to perform Box Jump Squats as much as possible, since that move is safer and lower in impact.

THE FOUR UPPER-BODY-INTENSIVE CARDIO MOVES

1. Mountain Climber
2. Donkey Kick
3. Break-Dancer
4. Chop

Here, too, you can use just about any upper-body pushing and pulling variation that you can perform quickly. Pushups and Rows, or Plyometric Pushups and Plyo Rows if you're fit enough, tend to work best. Most people don't have the strength, power, and conditioning needed to perform Pullups or Handstand Pushups quickly and for lots of reps. You could perform Jumping Pullups or Squat Pulls, if you'd like, as the lower-body assistance makes them doable.

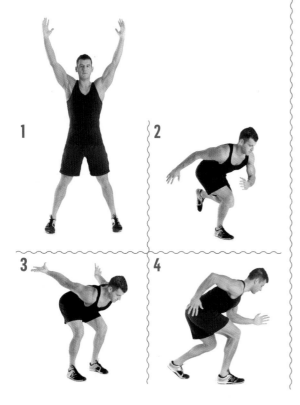

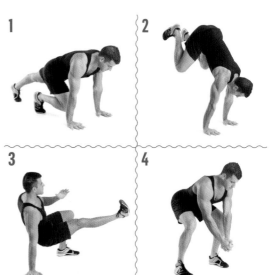

1. JUMPING JACK

This classic calisthenics cardio exercise is super simple to do, it works your whole body, and it's relatively low impact compared to other explosive exercises.

Stand with your feet together and your arms at your sides. Simultaneously jump your feet out to the side and bring your arms overhead, or as far overhead as you can pain free, based on your shoulder mobility. When in doubt, do a SEAL Jack; just bring your arms straight out to your sides, as that's plenty of motion without putting your shoulders in a tough position. Reverse the movement and repeat.

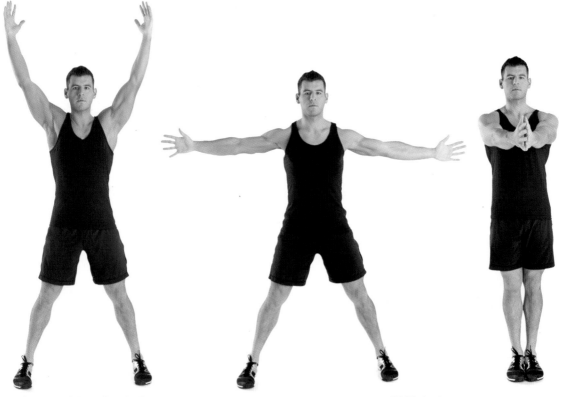

Overhead Jumping Jack   **SEAL Jack**

Focus more on turnover, getting out and back as quickly as you can, rather than jumping height, and stay on the balls of your feet throughout the movement. If you find this to be too difficult, modify the movement by stepping one foot out at a time to the same side with the same arm action to make it easier on your lower body. You can even eliminate the leg action altogether and just do the arm movement if you've suffered a lower-body injury.

Jumping Jacks can get boring. Here are three ways to juice your Jacks:

Variations

1. Change Arm and/or Foot Position

Cross your arms in front of your body at chest level. This better engages and stretches your chest and rear shoulder muscles and tends to be the preferred option for people with a history of shoulder pain. You can also cross your feet (a). Another option is moving your arms and feet forward and backward like you're cross-country skiing (b).

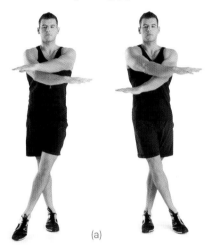

(a)

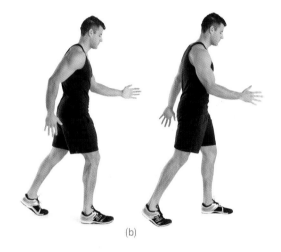

(b)

2. Involve a Squat

Drop your hips into a squatting motion to fire up your thighs and increase the difficulty. You can either start with your feet wide and bring them close together as you drop into a Squat (pictured) or start with your feet close and move them out wide to the side as you drop into a Squat.

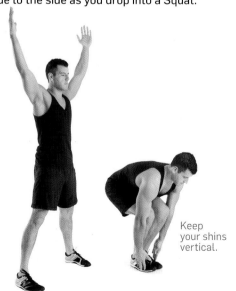

Keep your shins vertical.

3. Try a Pushup Jack

From the top of a Pushup position (or straight-arm Plank), jump your feet out and back without moving your hands.

MAKE IT HARDER: Get into a close-grip Pushup position with legs together as shown. Then jump both your hands and feet out and drop into the down position. Explosively push yourself airborne to bring your hands and feet back together in the top position.

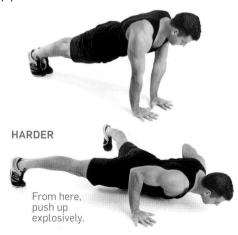

HARDER

From here, push up explosively.

2. SKATER JUMP

Like sprinting, jumping variations train total-body power. Jumping side to side will activate your fast-twitch muscle fibers, crush calories, and boost your heart rate as well as bulletproof your knees. Simply jump laterally from one foot to the other. Start with small (6-inch) jumps and work up to lateral leaps of 2 feet or more. For all of the progressions you must:

- Land with bends in your ankles, knees, and hips; get your butt back; and keep your back flat.

- Swing your arms across your body in the same direction of your jump.

- First stick each landing for 1 to 2 seconds before progressing to continuous jumps.

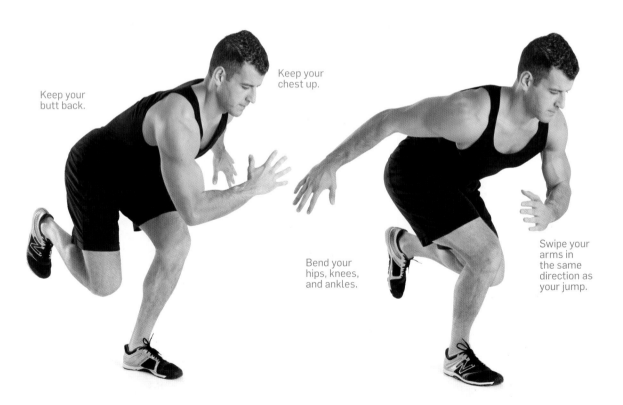

Keep your butt back.

Keep your chest up.

Bend your hips, knees, and ankles.

Swipe your arms in the same direction as your jump.

Variations

1. Skater Step

Step to one side and cross your trailing leg behind your body so that the foot makes contact with the ground. This provides two points of contact and more support and stability when jumping from one foot to the other. Repeat in the opposite direction.

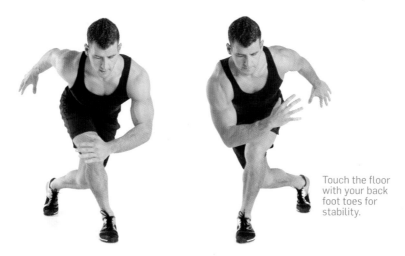

Touch the floor with your back foot toes for stability.

2. Rotational Skater Jump

This variation adds a rotational component in which you open up your hips and step back as you jump from one leg to the other. Then reverse the movement, switch sides, and repeat.

From standing, jump 90 degrees right, then back to the middle.

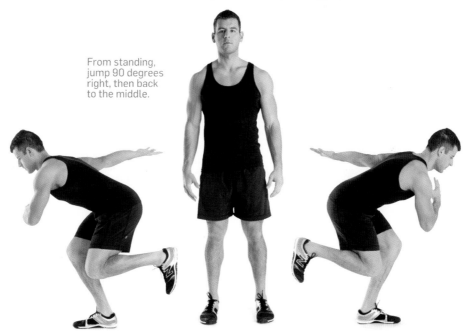

THE BODYWEIGHT 8 CARDIO EXERCISES 245

IIII 3. SKIER SWING

The Skier Swing offers the same benefit of a Kettlebell Swing without needing to swing a cannonball between your legs. It's called a Skier Swing because your body resembles that of a downhill skier when you hinge at your hips and reach your arms back behind your body. The move has all of the same elements as a Vertical Jump except your feet never leave the ground as you extend your arms overhead. This makes it lower impact and an excellent choice for higher reps. Internally rotate your arms when reaching back, with the thumbs turned in and the palms facing up. This puts your shoulders in the most stable position when your arms are behind your body. The majority of the movement occurs through the hips, though a little bit of bending at the knees is cool. Just make sure not to round your spine in the bottom position or hyperextend your lower back in the top position.

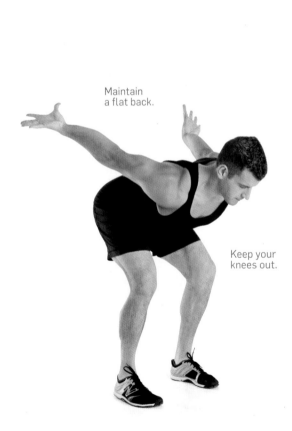

Maintain a flat back.

Keep your knees out.

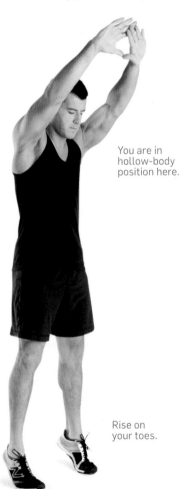

You are in hollow-body position here.

Rise on your toes.

Variation

Staggered Skier Swing

You can switch up your stance from a parallel stance to a staggered stance with the toes of the trailing foot aligned with the heel of the leading leg. This shifts more of the work to the hip of your leading leg. Make it even harder by performing Skier Swings while on only one leg at a time. You'll have to go a little slower because of the increased balance requirements.

To get the desired metabolism-boosting and calorie-burning effect, you'll need to perform Skier Swings with lots of speed and intention to make up for the fact that you're not holding on to any weights. Speed of movement is the great equalizer!

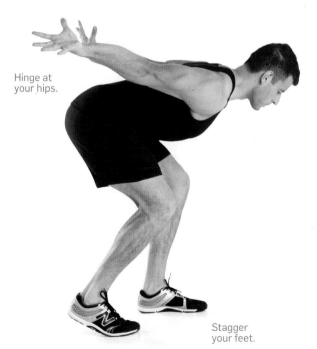

Keep your palms up with your thumbs pointing toward the ceiling.

Hinge at your hips.

Stagger your feet.

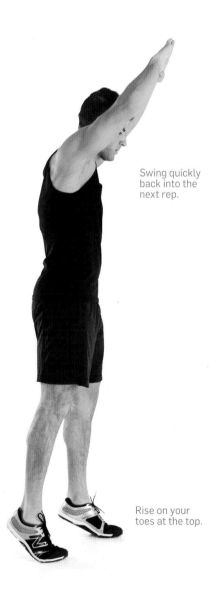

Swing quickly back into the next rep.

Rise on your toes at the top.

4. SPRINTER

Everyone knows that sprinting is a killer way to burn belly fat and get into crazy-good shape. But most people either aren't in good enough shape to sprint or don't have enough space to do so when at home or traveling. If you live in a northern climate, like I do in Milwaukee, then sprinting outdoors in winter just isn't happening unless you play for the Green Bay Packers. This exercise is your answer.

From a standing position, step your right leg back, hinge at your hips, and reach your right hand to the instep of your left or leading foot. Your back should remain flat. Briefly pause, then explosively step forward. Instead of going back to a full stand, you just go back and forth between the backward step and forward step, with the foot of one leg never leaving the ground. Pause and hold each position briefly before exploding back and forward as fast as you can. This variation emphasizes the start and drive phase of a sprint from a Sprinter stance. It's hip dominant and really targets the glutes and hamstrings. Perform all reps before switching legs.

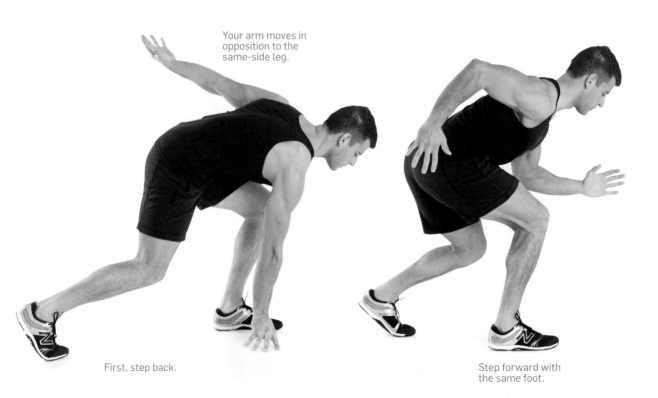

Your arm moves in opposition to the same-side leg.

First, step back.

Step forward with the same foot.

Variation

Sprinter Lunge

This variation emphasizes the stride phase of a sprint as your torso is more upright and your legs form 90-degree angles with the ground. It involves greater bending at the knees so it works your thighs better. In essence, you are adding the opposite arm–leg running action to a Reverse Lunge. As you step back into the bottom of a Reverse Lunge with your trailing knee hovering just above the floor, the hand opposite your leading leg should drive forward. As you pull your hips forward to stand up, you will lift the knee of your back leg while driving the opposite arm forward. Hold this position briefly, then reverse the movement and repeat with the foot of your leading leg never leaving the floor. Perform all of your reps on the same side before switching. You can make it harder by adding a jump to the top of the movement so that your leading leg leaves the floor momentarily before returning in preparation for the next Reverse Lunge.

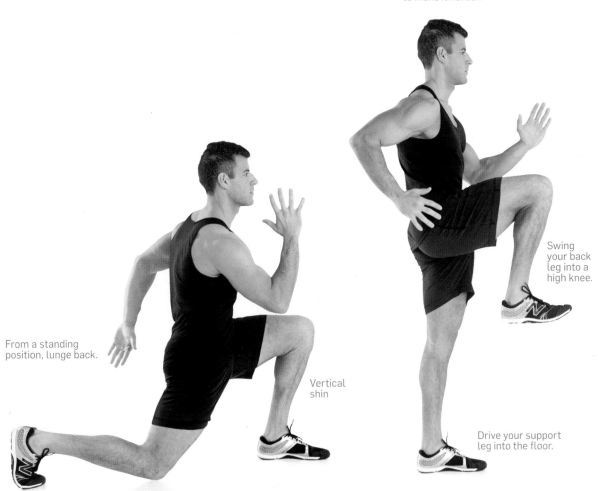

Add a hop at the top to make it harder!

Swing your back leg into a high knee.

From a standing position, lunge back.

Vertical shin

Drive your support leg into the floor.

Your back should form a straight line from knee, through hips to shoulders.

5. MOUNTAIN CLIMBER

When most people do Mountain Climber, the butt is piked way up in the air, the nose is in the ground, and the legs are sprawling all over like a bad '90s dance move.

The Mountain Climber is a great dynamic core-stability exercise, but you first need to master the static Pushup Hold or Plank position before you can do it with proper form. Keep your arms straight with your hands directly underneath your shoulders while also maintaining a straight-body position from head to toe. From this Plank starting position, drive your right knee toward your chest and touch that foot to the floor. As you straighten your right leg back, drive your left knee forward. Continue alternating legs in a climbing fashion as fast as you can with proper form. Done right, your hips move, not your lower back.

You can make Mountain Climbers easier by placing your hands on an elevated surface like a box, step, bench, chair, couch, or ottoman. Make them harder by adding a Pushup before every rep.

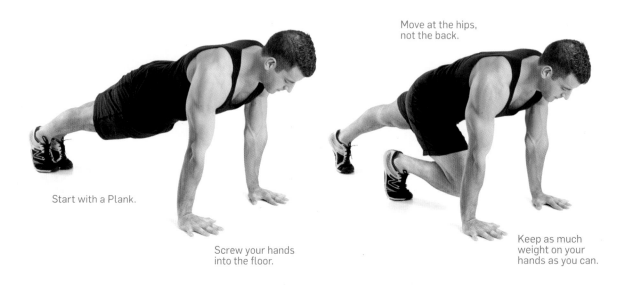

Start with a Plank.

Screw your hands into the floor.

Move at the hips, not the back.

Keep as much weight on your hands as you can.

Variations

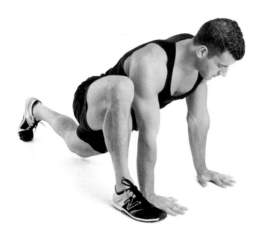

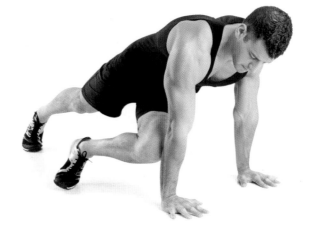

1. Spider Mountain Climber
Move one foot just outside the same-side hand, switch sides, and repeat.

2. Cross-Body Mountain Climber
Rotate your hips and upper back as you move one knee to the opposite elbow, switch sides, and repeat.

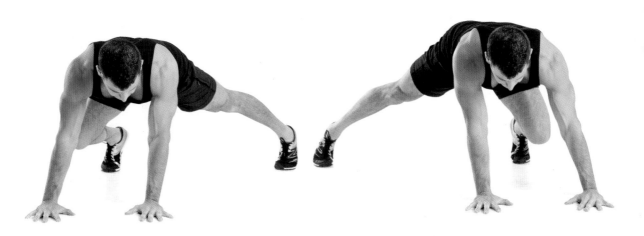

3. Side-to-Side Mountain Climber
Jump both feet from side to side and repeat.

6. DONKEY KICK

Some of the most effective bodyweight exercises are primal, resembling animal movements. You've crab-walked and duck-walked before, so you know these moves involve your entire body and are incredibly metabolic. Well, one of the best is the Donkey Kick. There are two distinct ways to set up for this ass-kicker:

Toes on the Floor: Place your hands flat on the floor with your knees bent at 90-degree angles, your feet directly underneath your hips, and your heels raised. This position should resemble the start of a Bear Crawl (see opposite page).

Feet Flat on the Floor (pictured): Hinge back at your hips and squat to place your hands down to the floor. Your back should be flat and feet flat on the floor. This position should resemble part of a Burpee. This requires more hip and ankle mobility.

Whatever starting position you use, the finish is the same. Place as much weight on your hands as possible. Lift your feet off of the floor and explosively extend your hips and legs as you kick behind your body. After your feet reach full extension, quickly bring your feet back to the starting position. Pause and reset for a moment and then repeat. A quick warning: Make sure there is no one or nothing behind you!

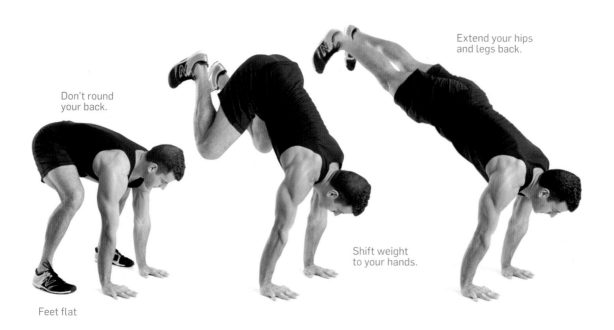

Don't round your back.

Extend your hips and legs back.

Shift weight to your hands.

Feet flat

Other Animal-Inspired Moves

1. Bear Crawl

Place your hands on the ground under your shoulders, get on your toes, and bend your knees, keeping them off the ground. Quickly move forward, backward, or laterally by moving the same-side hand and foot and following with the opposite hand and foot as a bear moves.

2. Crab Walk

You should be face up with your feet flat on the floor in front of you, your knees bent, and your hands on the floor under your shoulders. Crab walk forward, backward, or laterally, working the backside of your body.

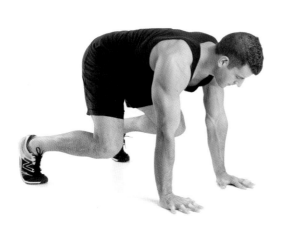

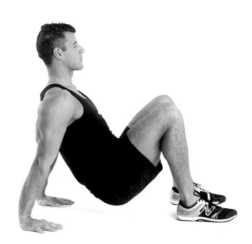

3. Crab Roll

This combines the Crab Walk and Bear Crawl into one exercise. Start in a Crab Walk position, pick up one hand and the opposite foot, and rotate your body to the Bear Crawl position. Reverse the movement, switch sides, and repeat.

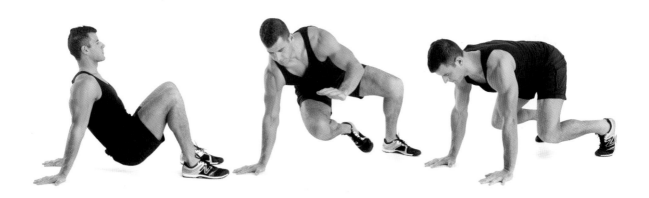

7. BREAK-DANCER

Breaking (or break-dancing) is an unreal test of bodyweight skills and conditioning. Like gymnastics, it takes years of dedicated practice and gradual progression to reach the levels of proficiency seen in real-deal breakers. It also takes some swagger.

But you can do it for exercise with no one looking. What I love about breaking is that it tests your upper-body and core strength and allows you to quickly move on your hands like you do on your feet. The key is to modify these movements so they can be safely performed in a state of serious fatigue. The best place to start is with a movement called the Lateral Kick-Through. Here's how to do it.

Assume a Pushup position with your knees bent at 90-degree angles and directly underneath your hips. This position should resemble the start of a Bear Crawl.

Rotate your body to the right and keep your left hand on the floor. Your right hand will come up off the floor and your left leg will swing underneath your body as you fully extend it to the right side. Notice how you pivot from the toes to a flat foot position on the supporting leg. Reverse the movement to come back to all fours, then switch sides and repeat. From here, add the variations on the opposite page.

Lateral Kick-Through

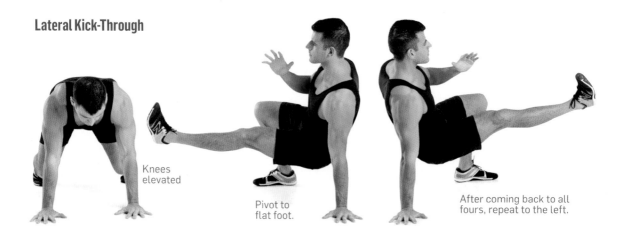

Knees elevated

Pivot to flat foot.

After coming back to all fours, repeat to the left.

Variations

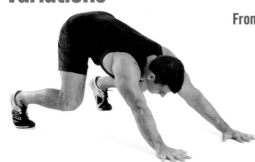

Front Kick-Through

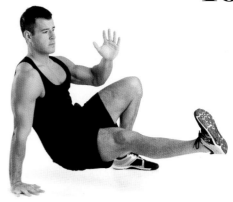

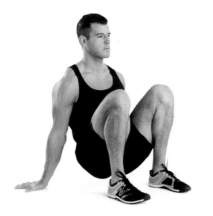

Pistol Switch

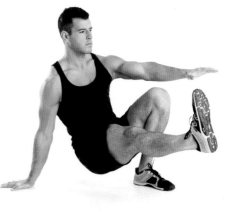

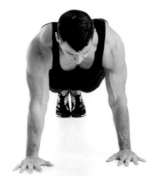

Breaker Planker 1

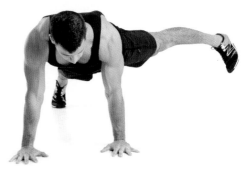

Breaker Planker 2

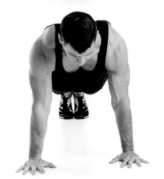

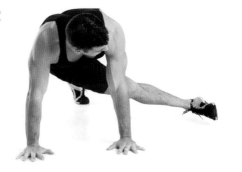

8. CHOP

Chopping has long been used to build core strength and improve cardio conditioning. It's often done while holding on to a medicine ball, using a cable pulling system, or even hitting a tire with a sledgehammer. Oh yeah, you can also chop wood with an ax. Clearly, none of that is gonna fly in a book about bodyweight exercises, though you could easily use a basketball or volleyball to replace the med ball, if you'd like. In the absence of an external load, all you need to do is increase speed of movement or decrease stability to keep challenging yourself. This way you can still chop off the chub without equipment.

Downward Chop

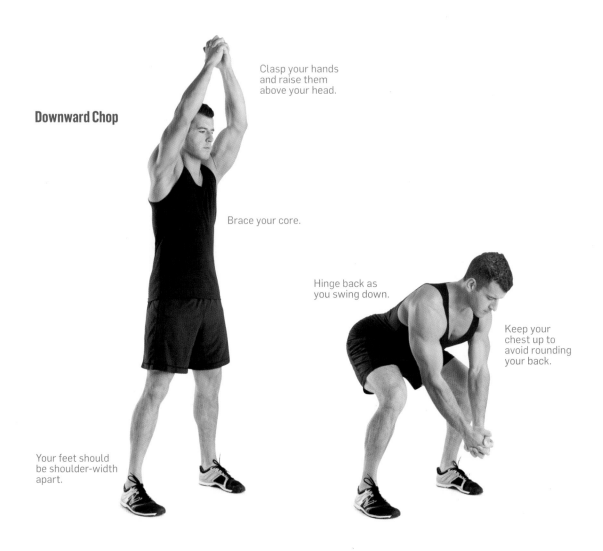

Clasp your hands and raise them above your head.

Brace your core.

Hinge back as you swing down.

Keep your chest up to avoid rounding your back.

Your feet should be shoulder-width apart.

Variations

Rotational Chop

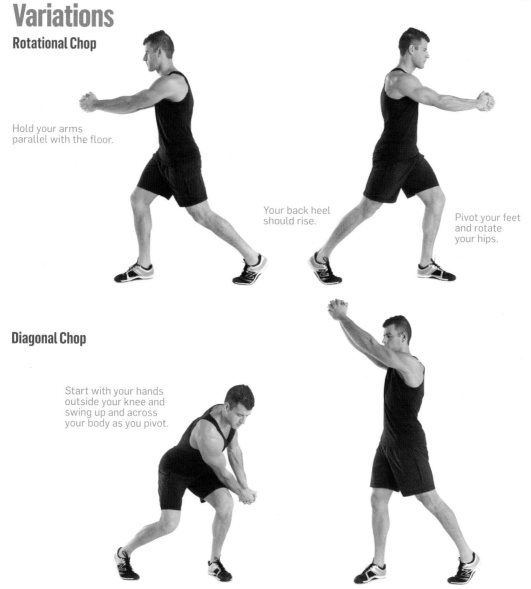

Hold your arms parallel with the floor.

Your back heel should rise.

Pivot your feet and rotate your hips.

Diagonal Chop

Start with your hands outside your knee and swing up and across your body as you pivot.

With all of the Chops, move your hips, not your lower back. When you're chopping down, drop your hips instead of rounding your spine. For Rotational or Diagonal Chops, you must pivot at your feet and rotate your hips to prevent any unwanted twisting of your lower back.

Once you can perform these exercises with speed and full range of motion from a parallel stance, progress to a split or staggered stance to challenge your core, hips, and knee stabilizers more. You can also squat down lower while chopping to make your thighs work harder. For all of the unilateral variations, be sure to perform an equal number of reps/sets on each side.

THE ULTIMATE BODYWEIGHT CARDIO WORKOUT

This workout is based on research that discovered that 20 seconds of maximum effort followed by 10 seconds of rest for eight total rounds (4 total minutes) resulted in greater fat loss and fitness improvements than 60 minutes of low- to moderate-intensity steady-state cardio. This research is well known as the Tabata study, which was done using stationary cycles. However, I've modified the workout in several ways. One, we're using functional bodyweight cardio exercises instead of a bike. Two, instead of doing the same exercise for all eight rounds, we're alternating between two noncompetitive exercises to keep intensity high and manage fatigue. Three, the workout is 20 total minutes to provide a larger direct calorie burn. If your goal is rapid fat loss, perform this cardio workout on off days between your Bodyweight Burners workouts (or strength workouts). Here's how it works.

There are four parts to this workout, each lasting 5 minutes.

In each part, you'll alternate between two bodyweight cardio moves, one that is lower-body intensive and the other upper-body intensive.

Perform 20 seconds of work for exercise 1 and then rest for 10 seconds. Then perform 20 seconds of work for exercise 2 and rest for 10 seconds. Repeat three more times, then rest a minute—that's 5 minutes. Then move to the next part of the workout.

If you'd prefer, you can perform all eight bodyweight cardio moves in one colossal cardio circuit; that is, you move from one exercise to the next after 1 set, and so on. Rest a minute after the eighth exercise and repeat up to three more times for a 20-minute workout.

❶ **Jumping Jack @ 20 seconds of work and 10 seconds of rest**

❷ **Mountain Climber @ 20 seconds of work and 10 seconds of rest**

❸ **Skater Jump @ 20 seconds of work and 10 seconds of rest**

❹ **Donkey Kick @ 20 seconds of work and 10 seconds of rest**

❺ **Skier Swing @ 20 seconds of work and 10 seconds of rest**

❻ **Break-Dancer @ 20 seconds of work and 10 seconds of rest**

❼ **Sprinter @ 20 seconds of work and 10 seconds of rest**

❽ **Chop @ 20 seconds of work and 10 seconds of rest**

For all unilateral exercises, switch sides at the halfway 10-second mark or from set to set.

MAKE IT EASIER: Modify the interval timeline to 15 seconds on, 15 seconds off, or even 10 seconds on, 20 seconds off.

MAKE IT HARDER: Cut the 10-second rest periods and immediately switch back and forth between the two moves for 4 straight minutes. Then rest a minute, move on to the next exercise pairing, and repeat up to three times for a 20-minute workout.

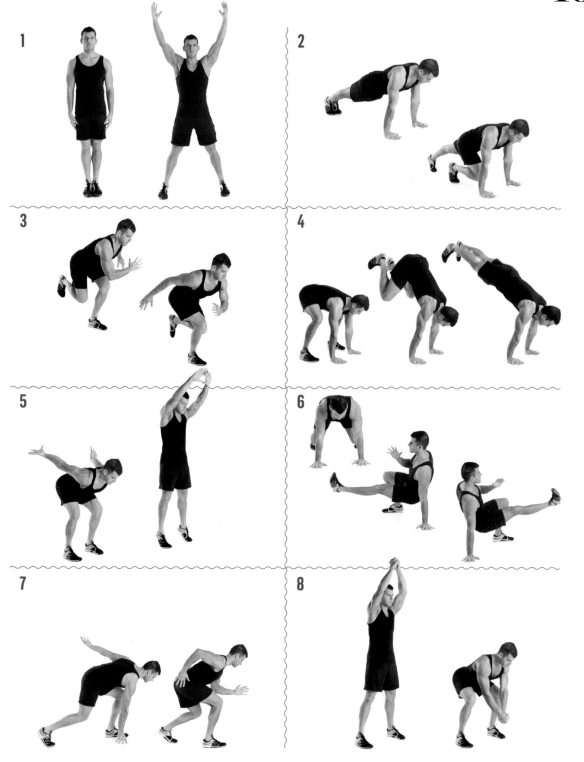

1

2

3

4

5

6

7

8

Acknowledgments

The more success I've been lucky to experience, the more I've realized how much help you need from good, selfless people along the way to live the life of your dreams. Here's a short list of the people who have lifted me up more than they'll ever know and ultimately made this book possible.

Thanks to my wife, Naomi, for being my best friend and most avid supporter over the years. We have been through a great deal together, and we keep getting better together, day by day, week by week, year by year. I look forward to lots more fun in our future. And thanks to you, I'm not even the best writer in my own house!

Thanks to *Men's Health* magazine and the Rodale family for the great honor of being able to represent your remarkable brand. I have been a reader of *MH* since my teens, and I still pinch myself every time I'm able to work with you in some way.

Thanks to Adam Campbell for being such a great mentor and providing me with the opportunity to be one of the featured fitness experts for the *Men's Health* brand. I truly admire your work ethic, creativity, and desire to make the fitness industry a better place. Thanks for giving me a shot.

Thanks to David Jack for introducing me to Adam and the amazing people at *Men's Health*. You are one of the most remarkable people I have ever met, and I look up to you more than words can describe. I hope that one day I will be able to make the same type of game-changing connection for someone else that you made for me.

Thanks to my investors in StreamFIT.com, who believed in me enough to support what was just a concept at the time. Together, we have built something out of nothing, and now people all over the world can work out with me and other top trainers anytime, anywhere without breaking the bank.

Thanks to my father, Brahim Gaddour, who came to this country with nothing but the hope of making a better life for his family. You taught me the value of hard work and gave me the discipline I needed to make the most out of what I've got. I'm forever grateful.

Thanks to my high school football coach, Don Forti, for introducing me to exercise. You made it fun, and you showed me the true power of fitness. Without your guidance, I doubt I would be doing what I do today. And I love what I do. Thanks, Coach!

Thanks to Jeff Csatari, my editor for this book, for working with me to create a blueprint for people to get in the best shape of their lives with nothing but their body weight. My gratitude also to the Rodale books team for all your talent and effort in producing this book.

Thanks to all of my former clients and boot campers for allowing me to hone my craft over the years. What I learned while working with you has made it possible for me to reach people all over the world. Without you, this book would not be possible.

Index

Boldface page references indicate photographs. <u>Underscored</u> references indicate boxed text and charts.

About the Author

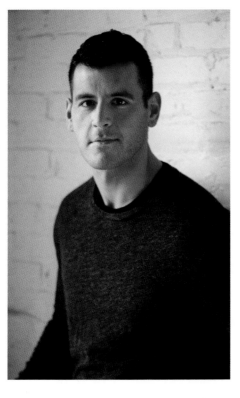

BJ Gaddour is a former fat kid with bum knees who transformed himself into one of *Men's Health* magazine's "100 Fittest Men of All Time." He is a certified strength and conditioning specialist (CSCS), a master of metabolic training, and an expert on bodyweight-only exercise.

Gaddour graduated from Amherst College in 2005. He went from working the front desk at a gym to owning a successful gym and then selling that same facility. He now consults with top fitness brands as a writer, speaker, featured fitness expert, on-camera talent, and fitness model.

Gaddour is the founder and CEO of StreamFIT, an online fitness resource that provides streaming workout videos for any device with Internet access. With hundreds of workouts featuring a wide variety of training styles, tools, intensities, and durations, StreamFIT is one of the most comprehensive fitness platforms available. For a free trial, visit StreamFIT.com.

He is also a regular contributor to *Men's Health* and *Women's Health* magazines and may be best known as the creator of the *Men's Health* DeltaFIT Speed Shred eight-DVD set and the *Men's Health* 10-Minute Torchers three-DVD set.

You can learn more about him at his blog (bjgaddour.com), where he shares fitness and nutrition tips with a little bit of comedy along the way. He currently lives in Milwaukee with his wife, Naomi, and their two boxers, Mustafa and Kaila.

The exercise DVDs *Bodyweight Cardio Burners* and *Bodyweight Muscle Burners*, which contain many of the exercises in this book, can be ordered at www.rodalestore.com/burners.html.